Mixed Martial Arts

The Beginners Guide to Mixed Martial Arts

(Unleashing the Power of Data Analytics in Mixed Martial Arts)

Lawrence Curtis

Published By **Elena Holly**

Lawrence Curtis

All Rights Reserved

Mixed Martial Arts: The Beginners Guide to Mixed Martial Arts (Unleashing the Power of Data Analytics in Mixed Martial Arts)

ISBN 978-1-7387533-3-8

No part of this guidebook shall be reproduced in any form without permission in writing from the publisher except in the case of brief quotations embodied in critical articles or reviews.

Legal & Disclaimer

The information contained in this book is not designed to replace or take the place of any form of medicine or professional medical advice. The information in this book has been provided for educational & entertainment purposes only.

The information contained in this book has been compiled from sources deemed reliable, and it is accurate to the best of the Author's knowledge; however, the Author cannot guarantee its accuracy and validity and cannot be held liable for any errors or omissions. Changes are periodically made to this book. You must consult your doctor or get professional medical advice before using any of the suggested remedies, techniques, or information in this book.

Upon using the information contained in this book, you agree to hold harmless the Author from and against any damages, costs, and expenses, including any legal fees potentially resulting from the application of any of the information provided by this guide. This disclaimer applies to any damages or injury caused by the use and application, whether directly or indirectly, of any advice or information presented, whether for breach of contract, tort, negligence, personal injury, criminal intent, or under any other cause of action.

You agree to accept all risks of using the information presented inside this book. You need to consult a professional medical practitioner in order to ensure you are both able and healthy enough to participate in this program.

Table Of Contents

Chapter 1: The Evolution of Combat Sports 1

Chapter 2: The Modern Era of Boxing 9

Chapter 3: The Rise of Modern MMA 16

Chapter 4: Training and Techniques....... 25

Chapter 5: MMA and the Beginning....... 33

Chapter 6: Equipment 46

Chapter 7: How to suit a mouthpiece 64

Chapter 8: MMA History 92

Chapter 9: Sparring Class 108

Chapter 10: Cleanliness........................ 131

Chapter 11: Talking and Horseplay 149

Chapter 12: Mental Preparation 165

Chapter 1: The Evolution of Combat Sports

Origins and History of Boxing

In the tremendous realm of fight sports sports sports activities, boxing stands as a cornerstone of area, abilties, and uncooked energy. Its roots may be traced returned hundreds of years to ancient civilizations that identified the innate human desire to interact in hand-to-hand fight. Let us embark on a journey via time, exploring the charming origins and ancient improvement of this noble paintings.

Around 3000 BCE, within the land of Sumer (cutting-edge-day-day Iraq), the earliest recorded proof of boxing emerged. Mesopotamian reliefs depicted fighters the use of their fists, showcasing the primitive form of the sport. These ancient bouts were likely a test of strength, agility, and courage, allowing individuals to display their prowess in a physical contest. The belief of fight as a method of self-expression and competition started out to take shape.

Fast forward to historical Greece, and boxing took on a more primarily based and ritualistic form because it have become an vital a part of the Olympic Games in 688 BCE. The Greeks, renowned for their appreciation of athletic prowess and bodily prowess, extended boxing to an art work form. They emphasized the significance of method and approach, recognizing that victory was no longer completely decided by means of using the usage of brute stress by myself. Athletes honed their talents through rigorous schooling, perfecting their footwork, stability, and protecting maneuvers.

To guard their hands within the direction of these intense encounters, the historic Greek boxers applied leather-based-based totally straps referred to as "himantes." These protecting coverings shielded their fists, allowing them to deliver effective blows with out preserving excessive accidents. Within the sacred grounds of the Olympic area, opposition would possibly step into the "pugme," a marked region specifically precise for boxing suits. Here, under the watchful eyes of masses of spectators, the pugilists engaged in a contest that examined their physical and intellectual fortitude.

The Romans, inspired via the usage of the Greek traditions, embraced boxing and added their very own versions. In Roman times, boxing fits frequently formed part of gladiatorial contests, wherein the roar of the gang mingled with the conflict of weapons and the grunts of fighters. To heighten the spectacle, boxers donned leather-based-based hand wraps known as "cestus." These shielding coverings were embedded with steel or spikes, transforming the sport proper right into a brutal display of energy and persistence. The combatants displayed terrific resilience as they absorbed and brought punishing blows.

However, with the autumn of the Roman Empire, organized boxing experienced a decline, leaving it dormant for loads of years. The remnants of this historic game ought to lay in wait, yearning for a resurgence.

The Renaissance of Boxing

In seventeenth-century England, boxing underwent a exceptional renaissance that might shape its modern-day form. It became in the course of this time that the sport began to adopt policies and hints, paving the way for its evolution proper right into a extra prepared and diffused area. Let us delve into the pivotal moments and influential figures that propelled boxing into a new technology.

In 1681, the game acquired a large beautify whilst champion fighter Jack Broughton introduced the primary recorded set of boxing regulations, referred to as the Broughton's Rules. These guidelines were a response to the growing concerns approximately the protection of contributors. Broughton sought to strike a balance a few of the uncooked depth of the sport and the need to shield the properly-being of the warring parties.

Broughton's Rules brought severa groundbreaking principles that revolutionized the game. One first rate component emerge as the use of padded gloves, which aimed to reduce the chance of severe accidents throughout bouts. This marked a shift a long way from the bare-knuckle brawls of the beyond.

Additionally, Broughton's Rules established the idea of rounds, ensuring that fights had been divided into manageable segments that allowed warring parties to get better and strategize among exchanges.

With the creation of these pointers, boxing fits were now achieved inner a roped-off place known as the hoop, presenting a controlled surroundings for the competition. The ring became a sacred region in which warriors clashed, their capability, power of mind, and resilience on entire show. The time period "ring" itself might turn out to be synonymous with the sport, representing the sacred vicinity wherein legends had been born and records become made.

Throughout the 18th and 19th centuries, boxing persisted to conform and benefit popularity. Bare-knuckle boxing have grow to be a defining aspect of the sport, characterized through excessive and grueling fights that captivated spectators. The appeal of witnessing two pugilists have interaction in a struggle of wills, relying on their naked fists and unwavering self-control, drew crowds from all walks of life. Champions like James Figg, Tom Cribb, and John L. Sullivan emerged as family names, taking pics the imaginations of the masses and etching their names into the annals of boxing records.

As boxing reached new heights, it faced its straightforward percentage of grievance and controversy. Detractors argued that the game modified into excessively violent, selling brutality and endangering the lives of the contributors. However, supporters of boxing countered the ones claims, putting forward that it became a testament to the human spirit and a exhibit of challenge, know-how, and resilience.

Chapter 2: The Modern Era of Boxing

The sunrise of the 20 th century delivered about extensive changes in the landscape of boxing. It modified right into a time of transformation, as the sport shed its raw and chaotic popularity to consist of a greater installation and managed technique. Let us discover the critical aspect dispositions that propelled boxing into the current generation.

One pivotal 2nd got here with the introduction of the Queensberry Rules in 1867. These regulations, named after the Marquess of Queensberry, aimed to refine and standardize the sport. They emphasized truthful play, sportsmanship, and the use of gloves, marking a departure from the bare-knuckle bouts that had characterized in advance iterations of boxing. The Queensberry Rules delivered a diploma of respectability and legitimacy to the game, paving the manner for its massive recognition.

The use of gloves not handiest reduced the threat of excessive accidents however additionally introduced a strategic detail to the bouts. Boxers had to adjust their strategies and approaches to house the presence of gloves, the usage of them as each offensive and protective system. The implementation of weight divisions further organized the game, permitting opponents to compete in opposition to warring parties of similar stature and talents.

As boxing persevered to comply, governing bodies at the side of the International Boxing Federation (IBF), World Boxing Association (WBA), and World Boxing Council (WBC) emerged as key gamers inside the law and advertising of the sport. These corporations oversaw championship bouts, mounted rankings, and ensured the adherence to rules and suggestions. They have end up the custodians of boxing's integrity, making sure sincere competition and imparting a platform for gifted warring parties to show off their skills on a worldwide diploma.

The contemporary-day technology of boxing introduced with it an terrific degree of worldwide recognition and fanfare. Iconic opponents along with Muhammad Ali, Joe Louis, and Mike Tyson transcended the boundaries of the game, fascinating audiences with their ability, air of mystery, and personal testimonies. Their exploits in the ring have end up the stuff of legend, as they battled bold combatants and etched their names within the records books.

The creation of television and the upward thrust of pay-in line with-view occasions catapulted boxing into the homes of tens of tens of millions worldwide. Fans eagerly tuned in to witness epic clashes, marveled on the high-quality footwork, devastating knockouts, and suggests of unwavering strength of will. World name fights have end up tremendous spectacles, drawing now not handiest boxing aficionados but also casual viewers who have been enthralled through manner of manner of the drama, pleasure, and unyielding spirit that boxing embodied.

In recent years, boxing has continued to captivate audiences and adapt to the wishes of the ever-changing global. New schooling strategies, scientific upgrades, and a heightened recognition on safety have reshaped the game. Promoters and executives tirelessly artwork to reveal off talented warring parties and offer enthusiasts with unforgettable bouts that ignite ardour and encourage awe.

As we mirror upon the wonderful journey of boxing, from its ancient origins to the grandeur of the contemporary-day technology, we witness a tapestry woven with memories of courage, resilience, and the unyielding pursuit of greatness. The statistics of boxing serves as a testomony to the indomitable human spirit, a celebration of functionality, method, and the pursuit of athletic excellence.

The Birth of Mixed Martial Arts

In the arena of fight sports activities, mixed martial arts (MMA) has emerged as a charming and dynamic area that mixes severa strategies from particular martial arts traditions. Let us embark on a journey to discover the origins and historical improvement of this thrilling combat interest, witnessing the evolution of MMA from its humble beginnings to its popularity as a international phenomenon.

The roots of MMA can be traced back to historical civilizations that recognized the need for bendy combat competencies. In historical Greece, the Olympic Games showcased a lot of fight sports sports, consisting of pankration, a blend of putting and grappling strategies. Pankration modified right into a fierce and excessive undertaking that tested the athletes' physical and highbrow fortitude, embracing a holistic technique to combat.

Throughout data, diverse cultures round the area advanced their personal hybrid martial arts systems, mixing elements of placing, wrestling, and submission strategies. For example, in Japan, the paintings of "shooto" blended wrestling and striking strategies, developing a dynamic and bendy fashion of combat.

However, it become not until the latter 1/2 of the twentieth century that the cutting-edge-day form of MMA started out to take shape. In Brazil, the Gracie own family performed a pivotal role inside the evolution of MMA via their development of Brazilian Jiu-Jitsu (BJJ). The Gracies, led through Helio Gracie and his sons, diffused their grappling techniques to overcome larger and stronger warring parties. Their dominance in challenge suits and early MMA competitions showcased the effectiveness of BJJ in actual-worldwide combat conditions.

Chapter 3: The Rise of Modern MMA

The Nineties marked a turning element within the records of MMA, as a series of activities and influential figures propelled the game into the mainstream. In 1993, the Ultimate Fighting Championship (UFC) have become set up, imparting a platform for fighters from numerous martial arts backgrounds to compete in opposition to each different in a controlled surroundings.

The early days of the UFC witnessed a clash of patterns, as combatants from disciplines along with boxing, kickboxing, wrestling, and Brazilian Jiu-Jitsu confronted off within the Octagon. These pioneering activities captivated audiences with their raw intensity and the spectacle of severa martial artists trying out their skills in the path of each other.

As the game received traction, competition and taking walks shoes realized the importance of being nicely-rounded and talented in multiple martial arts disciplines. The idea of "blended martial arts" emerged, emphasizing the want to be flexible and adaptable as a way to succeed inside the ever-evolving landscape of combat sports activities.

Over the years, the tips and policies of MMA have been touchy to prioritize fighter protection and promote sincere opposition. Striking strategies, grappling maneuvers, and submission holds have been blended, developing a dynamic and interesting fashion of fight. Fighters professional in more than one disciplines, honing their capabilities in placing arts like boxing, Muay Thai, and taekwondo, in addition to grappling arts like Brazilian Jiu-Jitsu and wrestling.

MMA within the Modern Era

As MMA received popularity, organizations together with Bellator MMA, ONE Championship, and Professional Fighters League (PFL) emerged, presenting systems for fighters to show off their competencies on a worldwide degree. These organizations hosted activities featuring top-ranked warring parties from round the sector, charming fanatics with their suggests of approach, athleticism, and coronary coronary coronary heart.

The increase of MMA has been in addition fueled through using improvements in media insurance and generation. Pay-in step with-view occasions, streaming offerings, and social media systems have enabled fans to get right of entry to stay fights and in the back of-the-scenes content material fabric cloth, developing a higher connection amongst warring parties and their supporters.

In cutting-edge years, MMA has transcended the location of endeavor and entered the nation-states of leisure and mainstream way of lifestyles. The emergence of charismatic and professional fighters on the side of Conor McGregor, Anderson Silva, Ronda Rousey, and Jon Jones has introduced the sport to new heights, fascinating audiences with their performances within the Octagon and their magnetic personalities outside of it.

Furthermore, MMA has come to be a international phenomenon, with events taking place in severa nations and attracting fighters from various backgrounds. The mission has embraced splendid patterns and strategies from round the sector, in addition enriching its tapestry of fight arts.

The origins of MMA can be traced lower lower returned to ancient civilizations that identified the need for flexible combat abilties. Through the a long time, hybrid martial arts structures and the pursuit of properly-rounded schooling paved the manner for the present day-day form of MMA.

From the early days of the UFC to the worldwide phenomenon it's miles nowadays, MMA has captivated audiences with its aggregate of putting, grappling, and submission techniques. The exercise keeps to conform, with opponents constantly pushing the limits of what's possible within the Octagon.

As we've got amusing the origins and increase of MMA, we apprehend the electricity of will, assignment, and expertise of the fighters who've propelled the sport to its modern-day-day stature. MMA embodies the spirit of competition, showcasing the high-quality physical and intellectual talents of its athletes.

The Intersection of Boxing and MMA

The Crossover Appeal

In the realm of fight sports activities sports, the worlds of boxing and combined martial arts (MMA) have intersected in a fascinating way. The collision of those disciplines has captivated audiences international, generating pleasure and showcasing the skills of warring parties who very own the potential to excel in each sports activities sports sports activities. Let us discover the thrilling relationship among boxing and MMA, witnessing the moments in which those extremely good worlds collide.

The crossover among boxing and MMA stems from the shared basis of putting. Both sports activities activities emphasize the art work of landing powerful punches and evading incoming attacks. The precision, timing, and footwork honed in boxing display to be valuable belongings for MMA combatants on the lookout for to excel in stand-up exchanges.

The enchantment of the crossover is twofold. For boxers, the venture of entering into the MMA arena offers an opportunity to check their competencies in competition to opponents who convey a numerous shape of techniques. It pushes them out in their consolation zones and forces them to conform to the intricacies of grappling and submission holds. Likewise, for MMA warring parties, the hazard to compete inside the boxing ring provides a hazard to show off their putting skills in a greater targeted and specialised surroundings.

The Boxing-MMA Superfights

Over the years, numerous immoderate-profile boxing-MMA superfights have captured the attention of lovers global.

These matchups function spectacles that skip beyond the boundaries of the individual sports activities activities, pitting mythical warring parties from different disciplines closer to each different. Let us delve into some of the most iconic encounters which have taken region at the intersection of boxing and MMA.

One of the most memorable crossovers took place in 2017 at the same time as boxing legend Floyd Mayweather Jr. Stepped into the ring to stand MMA movie star Conor McGregor. The matchup generated splendid hype and anticipation, because the arena of boxing collided with the region of MMA. Mayweather's tremendous boxing skills had been pitted in the direction of McGregor's unorthodox setting fashion. The occasion captivated audiences, showcasing the capability of waft-vicinity matchups and illustrating the perfect demanding situations faced through fighters transitioning from one game to every extraordinary.

In modern years, more boxers and MMA opponents have explored the opportunity of trying out their abilities within the path of disciplines. The likes of Anderson Silva, a former UFC middleweight champion, stepped into the boxing ring, showing his placing prowess in the direction of famend boxers. Similarly, MMA fighter Ben Askren faced off toward YouTuber-became-boxer Jake Paul, drawing interest from every MMA and boxing enthusiasts.

These crossover superfights provide a platform for athletes to reveal off their versatility and pass beyond the limits of their respective sports activities activities. They ignite debates and discussions, fueling the creativeness of fanatics and upsetting desires of what may be feasible whilst the worlds of boxing and MMA collide.

Chapter 4: Training and Techniques

The intersection of boxing and MMA has no longer handiest sparked high-profile superfights but has moreover inspired the training and strategies hired with the useful resource of opponents in every disciplines. As MMA opponents are looking for to enhance their putting competencies, they turn to the instructions of boxing to enhance their footwork, precision, and shielding talents.

Boxing schooling techniques, which includes shadow boxing, heavy bag artwork, and attention mitt drills, have located their vicinity in the education wearing occasions of MMA opponents. The situation and precision instilled in boxing schooling help MMA opponents expand the placing skills crucial to succeed within the Octagon.

Likewise, the incorporation of things from MMA into boxing education has brought a modern-day measurement to the candy technology. The have a look at of takedown safety, clinch paintings, and techniques for handling various putting patterns has advanced the repertoire of boxers, allowing them to adapt to big situations and fighters.

The intersection of boxing and MMA continues to encourage combatants to push the bounds in their capabilities and discover new opportunities. This skip-pollination of strategies and training techniques enriches the arsenal of fighters in both sports activities activities, developing properly-rounded athletes who can excel in numerous fight situations.

The intersection of boxing and MMA represents a fascinating and evolving relationship among outstanding however interconnected combat sports sports. The crossover between the two disciplines gives fighters the threat to test their competencies, captivate audiences, and push the boundaries of what is viable within the ring and the Octagon.

As boxing and MMA hold to thrive and evolve, we are able to anticipate more crossover superfights, new training methodologies, and an ongoing change of strategies. The collision of these worlds gives a thrilling spectacle that showcases the resilience, abilties, and flexibility of the athletes involved.

Beyond the Ring and Octagon

Boxing and mixed martial arts (MMA) have transcended the world of sports activities and entered the geographical regions of enjoyment, well-known culture, or even style. The impact of those combat sports activities sports sports activities extends some distance beyond the ring and the Octagon, permeating severa components of society and capturing the creativeness of people throughout the arena. Let us discover the effect of boxing and MMA on well-known way of life, witnessing how those sports have grow to be cultural phenomena.

One of the most extraordinary techniques wherein boxing and MMA have impacted famous manner of existence is through the upward push of iconic warring parties who have end up family names. Legends consisting of Muhammad Ali, Mike Tyson, and Conor McGregor have transcended their sports sports sports, becoming cultural icons whose have an impact on extends past their athletic achievements. Their large-than-lifestyles personalities, fascinating performances, and memorable charges have made them symbols of power, resilience, and determination, inspiring generations of fanatics.

Moreover, the sports activities of boxing and MMA have been featured in numerous films, television suggests, and documentaries, further solidifying their presence in well-known way of life. Films like "Rocky" and "Million Dollar Baby" have end up iconic representations of the human spirit and the pursuit of greatness in boxing. Similarly, MMA-themed movies which consist of "Warrior" and "Never Back Down" have captivated audiences, showcasing the depth and drama of the game.

Fashion and Style

Another location wherein boxing and MMA have left their mark is the world of style and fashion. The have an impact on of opponents' apparel, from boxing robes to MMA fight shorts, has permeated mainstream fashion, with human beings donning these iconic portions as a photo of electricity and self guarantee. The aesthetics of combat sports activities, characterised through ambitious shades, placing designs, and the instance of fighter manufacturers, have grow to be well-known in streetwear and athletic clothing.

Furthermore, the frame and education strategies of boxers and MMA warring parties have stimulated health trends and frame ideals. The choice to obtain a robust, lean, and athletic body has led many humans to embody schooling techniques stimulated through those fight sports activities. Fitness applications and lessons that incorporate elements of boxing and MMA have received reputation, permitting fanatics to experience the bodily and highbrow benefits of these disciplines.

Inspiring Stories and Philanthropy

Boxing and MMA have moreover served as structures for inspiring reminiscences of conquer adversity and acts of philanthropy. From rags-to-riches narratives to fighters using their platform to make a pleasant impact, those sports activities sports have showcased the resilience, strength of will, and compassion in their athletes.

Many combatants have come from humble beginnings, overcoming annoying conditions and obstacles to gain the top in their respective sports sports. Their memories of perseverance and strength of will resonate with audiences, inspiring them to pursue their personal goals and overcome their very non-public struggles.

Additionally, combatants have used their reputation and achievement to provide lower lower back to their agencies and make a difference in the world. Whether through charitable foundations, network outreach applications, or the usage of their platform to raise popularity for social reasons, boxers and MMA opponents have installed a self-control to growing a pleasing effect beyond their athletic endeavors.

Chapter 5: MMA and the Beginning

When I began out my look for a MMA or grappling faculty the closest was 100 and fifty miles away. So armed with the contemporary information I had from seasoned wrestling I commenced out adapting what I knew. I although persisted my look for any sort of schooling I might also want to get my palms on. One of my preferred combatants of the time, Ken Shamrock had published a e-book called Inside the Lion's Den. This gave me an belief to how a MMA university turn out to be run. I felt a kinship with him, from every of our pro wrestling backgrounds. After I sold his Lion's Den e-book, I commenced out setting collectively my organization. This is also my first foray into running a school/organization. In the start it end up simply my pals and me getting together, working out and studying. This is also as soon as I got here to my first awareness approximately being a university proprietor or strolling a group. My very first lesson turn out to be very hardly ever is all people as reliable or committed to this as you the school proprietor/educate. I determined speedy that I became the guy that become usually going to be there. I grow to be the man that showed up no matter what the weather have grow to be like or regardless of what have become taking location. I became lucky currently my dad owned the fitness center and I sincerely took up some location within the lower once more. If I had to pay the bills I might were closed in the first month. I determined out speedy that no character is probably as dedicated to my university as I became. It took me a while to research that no student will be as dedicated to the university as me. By all way be there on your college students, however don't lose sight of the significance of your own family. Be there for them too.

Never the a lot much less I continued. I even have become nonetheless in love with grappling and MMA. I persevered to seek out one-of-a-kind belongings of training, and on the equal time I began training a bit extra officially on the gymnasium. I become now schooling a MMA class multiple nights every week and schooling a pro wrestling class multiple nights each week. I turn out to be slowly deciding on up some university students with a few determination. MMA in Missouri became ultimately starting to capture up with the west coast. The first authentic MMA display modified into held in Columbia MO. I myself had already been doing a little non sanctioned fights at pro wrestling indicates and at gyms. Grappling tournaments were furthermore beginning to be greater not unusual. We now had an outlet, a place to exhibit the hard paintings we were doing. I now had guys competing so it modified into time to get our act collectively. We had no actual idea on what to do. I continued to are seeking out any statistics that I need to. YouTube have end up now not an possibility proper now, so books and those were my greatest resources of records. I tried to pick out up as plenty as I have to from any supply. I emulated colleges just like the Lion's Den. We had system, a 10' x 10' mat to begin and later a 20' x 20', an area, and the willingness to art work difficult and chase our dreams.

Coaching and Competing in MMA

Let's start with a check listing of factors you may need to do and to have if you want to compete or be an MMA Coach. There are topics that may not be on this listing don't be afraid to feature your non-public personal touches. This is a excellent start and will manual you within the proper route.

Consistent Training

It is viable to compete in case you most effective teach some nights each week, however it will likely be tough to compete at the better levels of MMA. Now this doesn't endorse you have to be in a MMA university six days in line with week. I believe to gain the know-how necessary to compete in MMA you want as a minimum three days of approach and endeavor particular training in line with week. Then you need at the least in some unspecified time within the future each week sparring. Then you may also want one to two days consistent with week jogging on aerobic and power education. This can be combined with one of the different days. It is also brilliant to exercising no extra than three to four days in a row, without an afternoon of rest in among. Of course you could harm your agenda up but works for you or the gymnasium you attend. BUT no more than three or 4 days in a row without a rest day.

Let me offer an purpose behind what I recommend via way of relaxation day in advance than the collective internet jumps on me. You can truly lie round and do not anything, but it's far usually awesome to perform a touch issue mild which will maintain you free and workout a few pain. Also a day exercises aren't 100% vital. A lot of pro warring parties do it this manner due to the fact it's miles a manner to them. They gets a commission to exercising consultation and fight. Most combatants I recognize novice or pro however have day jobs. This limits the two an afternoon training extensively. But do no longer lose coronary coronary heart it can even though be finished. The first trouble is be regular. Your teach will thank you, your teammates will thanks, and your performance on fight night time time will thank you.

Coaching

You ought to have the proper humans to help you to your journey. It is form of impossible to gain the abilties you need to your personal. I have turn out to be not able to sincerely take region all of the talents I needed to teach or combat on my own, I had to find out the records and get the training. Now days you can discover an entire lot of information at the net, DVDs, and books. This is a outstanding manner to investigate, but in the long run if you need to be right you need to discover a teach. They are available.

If you have got the danger go to different faculties, go to the community MMA fights and note how the guys do from unique gyms. Look for professionalism. A lot of instances you may in fact watch how the combatants act inside the cage. Listen to the coaches within the corner. Are they clearly giving instructions? Are they giving their fighter path, or are they sincerely yelling hit'em. This is a useless deliver away of a educate to live far from. Talk to close by promoters, maximum will steer you in a quite accurate course. They are used to managing combatants and coaches. They will inform you which of them of them ones ones to looking for out and which ones to keep away from in any respect fees.

Fighters don't commonly make the tremendous coaches, so don't expect honestly due to the truth a educate does now not have a seasoned fight career, he might no longer make an wonderful train. Look at his warring parties. See how they act and the manner they carry out. Do they act like specialists? Do they appear like knowledgeable expert warring parties? I've watched sufficient network MMA over the years to inform you the guys that do not have a solid teach stand out like a sore thumb.

On the opposite issue of that, if you need to be a teach, it approach which you need to be open and studies as an entire lot as possible. You want to be able to deliver your guys that method to most all in their questions, put together schooling camps, and activity plans for fights. If you need to stand out act professional and appearance expert.

Location

Guys located some of emphasis on locating a building and starting a university. Now once I started out out I actually have come to be lucky, I had a place wherein I didn't have to fear about the bills. Now this is incredible for peace of thoughts however does now not something for making me a higher enterprise guy. Truthfully all you want is some mat region, a piece little little bit of device, an great educate or education capabilities, and willingness to have a look at. You don't should have a multimillion greenback facility. Cause frankly till you're famous or wealthy it's going to maximum in all likelihood not be successful. I'm not pronouncing this to scare anybody from following their dream. If your dream is to personal an exquisite faculty without a doubt be practical whilst beginning. Start modest and allow your abilties as a train, increase. As your competencies develop and additionally you turn out to be higher, it'll display. This will help bring together your organization. Now in case you are a fighter and feature get admission to to an area like this with appropriate education you have to be there already. Here is the trouble with small rural areas like in which I'm from, those locations don't exist. This became definitely the hassle I had after I began. This is the precept cause I began getting to know on my own faculty

No vicinity to move. Let's have a take a look at what is going on in recent times, especially with amateur MMA. You commonly have two or 3 real exceptional schools indoors a fifty mile radius. These colleges have all the equipment you want to fight at an novice degree and perhaps a pro degree. Then you have a collection of schools that are not continually the satisfactory. They are usually in a person's storage or basement. Now this isn't a trouble if you have a very good train and gadget. But commonly if there is a superb coach and the proper system we would no longer even embody them in the 2d price schools. Truthfully you really can not name them schools. They are normally product of some guys who get collectively and educate on and rancid. Again if this is what you're presently doing, this is top notch, but in case you need to transport as lots as the subsequent degree you want to have a educate, and if you are the educate ensure you have end up the skills had to get your guys palms raised. Let me stress this, training does now not suggest getting together together along side your pals and sparring like maniacs for a couple of hours. If all you're doing is sparring you are performing some component incorrect. Whether you're a fighter or a teach, there need to be some studying involved. Yes you can studies things from sparring. But sparring is the software of the things you study. Sparring is a time to tweak and great song, no longer placed the tough pressure within the laptop.

Location does no longer commonly endorse greatness. Go visit the college see if it suits you and your desires. If you've got were given a college in your garage or basement, make sure you're schooling your guys the proper way. Even no matter the fact that this section is set college location if all you're doing is sparring you are not a school. School is for learning.

Chapter 6: Equipment

So some distance we've got got decided that region is not a deal breaker, but having a train is. Let's communicate approximately device. You best ought to have some pieces of clearly mandatory system. The first piece of tool you need being a mat of some type. Now the number one mat I had have become a 10 x 10 wrestling mat. This changed into handiest massive sufficient for two guys to be on at a time however it served its reason. So a mat is a obligatory requirement everywhere you teach.

Next may be some form of heavy bag. It can be just a conventional heavy bag, a banana muay thai bag, or maybe a flowery tear drop bag. One element to make sure of is that it can be eliminated from the ceiling. It can be a useful tool for working at the floor. We have mat and heavy bag, next may be. No wait that is truly all of your education vicinity has to have. Even in case your health club or university has now not anything extra than a mat and a heavy bag you could be suitable to go. When I had my MMA gymnasium going I had a mat vicinity, a cage, weight vicinity, and a boxing ring multi function constructing. This have come to be a first rate setup, however it wasn't a one hundred% important. Mat and heavy bag is all you want.

If you're clearly setting up a university, here is in which you can positioned your initial device buy into. You might likely want to carry out a chunk looking for to discover a few low-price, however they may be obtainable. In this financial device it looks like more faculties are final than putting in. If you have got a college that offers MMA as a category and no longer actually grappling you will want a few manner to art work on the cage. This can be a cage itself. They do make a few very small ones for gyms, and some that absolutely sit down proper on your mat. You can get a cage panel and mount it on the wall to your mat. Or you may have a padded wall. You will want this type of to clearly art work on what makes a cage so unique than fighting in a hoop or simply on a mat. The cage panel does have a touch deliver to it, but for the most element it is a sturdy wall. As a fighter it can be a terrific weapon or a big criminal responsibility if you don't understand a way to do cope with it. It is part of being a mma fighter, similar to being able to field or conflict. If you have got more pads all you want to do is mount them on the wall. Velcro works super for this. It obtained't destroy your padding and it shouldn't destroy the wall. I might make one notion is if you have drywall covered partitions I could endorse putting in more than one sheets of plywood behind your mats. That want to hold absolutely everyone from pulling a juggernaut and strolling through the wall.

If you have got a person accessible with a welder you can make a pretty proper duration cage panel from 1x1 steel tube and included chain hyperlink fence. You can order the chain link from most domestic development shops. Then weld up a body similar to the immoderate greenback cage panels you notice at unique gyms, mount it to the wall and you're in organisation. If you are difficult pressed to find out some padding in your new cage panel, try foam swim noodles. Slice it proper down the center and you may stick it proper on there with a piece tape. The addition of a cage panel or padded wall will make all of the difference within the great of instruction and fighters coming out of a health club. There is not any manner to simulate takedowns off the cage panel without some factor to put men towards. Please do not use galvanized chain hyperlink fence. It can be murder on you and your men. There is a reason they use lined chain hyperlink fence. This may be hard on you too. I continuously pick out best a matted wall.

Personal Equipment

The next component is personal tool. For MMA you need gloves, MMA and boxing. Wait boxing gloves. Yes boxing gloves. I had a thirty minute communique with a pupil not too long in the beyond approximately why we want boxing gloves. Most human beings should assume this a given, however allow's ruin it down. You can not spar with five ounce gloves. At least no longer at the level you can spar with boxing gloves. Yes you could spar with MMA gloves and we are able to move over an appropriate and realistic way to spar with MMA and boxing gloves. It truely does not bode well in your face if you are sparring difficult.

There are a ton of diverse patterns and weights of gloves on hand. So here's a short compare for gloves and glove weights. Boxing gloves which may be used for sparring have to be at least 14oz or 16oz, MMA gloves that are used for sparring should be no smaller than 6oz, 5oz if it's far a totally controlled sparring session. If you're competing in beginner MMA is also suitable to have a tough and rapid of competition gloves. This is because of the fact all promotions or sanctioning our bodies protective beginner MMA do no longer continuously offer gloves for competition. This is a few problem we are capable of cover in a later bankruptcy at the same time as we talk about competing in MMA.

Now again to the gloves. MMA gloves aren't for protecting your fighters head.

They are for defensive your fingers from his face, and granted they will be no longer the outstanding for that. If you observe a boxing glove and MMA glove and you trust you studied how is this going to protect my hand. Here is the argument I've commonly heard approximately MMA gloves. First warring parties do now not punch as difficult with MMA gloves to protect their palms. Well that is a bunch of BS. All the men I realize and myself protected by no means had that concept even move their thoughts except a hand have become injured. Then you still needed to punch the fellow a dozen times earlier than your thoughts says hiya stop it. Here is one which I even have additionally heard masses. You don't get the pinnacle trauma that you do with boxing gloves. I do now not take transport of as genuine with this constantly has loads to do with gloves and extra to do with the sports activities activities themselves. Boxers commonly combat 10-12 three minute rounds. MMA is generally three or 5 rounds of three to 5 mins, depending on novice or expert. Boxing has a status 8 depend. MMA does no longer. So you've got recuperation time in a boxing in shape. MMA you do not. MMA you get knocked down you will maximum probably have man sitting for your chest dropping hammers for your head from mount. Boxers spend a ton of time studying a way to take punches and reduce effect. They learn how to experience punches and slip punches. This is because of the truth the best weapon is punching your opponent. But you still get more head trauma due to the fact considered one of your important goals in boxing is to reboot your opponent's pc. Turn their mind off, KO. Boxers commonly put on a 10-sixteen ounce glove relying on education or opposition.

So take equal men placed a 5 ounce glove on him then a sixteen ounce glove on the opportunity, and you display the felony suggestions of physics accurate. Bigger glove more difficult punch. Ok permit me make clean this with one greater element I actually have heard due to the truth the start of MMA gloves. MMA gloves reason extra superficial damage than boxing gloves, so they are more stable. Well that is one manner to check it. The game just isn't vintage sufficient to sincerely see the long time effects of getting punched within the head with the smaller glove. I do realise on every occasion you are taking a punch to the pinnacle it motives harm now not rely what kind of glove. I don't want to scare absolutely everyone from doing MMA due to the reality I love the game, but the reality is with combat sports activities sports you may go through some form of thoughts harm if you get punched in the head. It won't be as a whole lot as if you were a boxer. That is simply the character of the most effective-of-a-kind sports. Boxers will continuously train to punch each wonderful in the head have been a mixed martial artist trains such pretty a few various things. Boxing isn't typically the main hobby. Just understand no matter what sort of glove, there are consequences for buying punched inside the head.

It does sound stupid but I started out to word variations in myself after getting my cage rattled a few instances whilst sparring. I comprehend I've had at least 4 or 5 concussions through the years, a few simply from sparring within the gym. Not to say, playing soccer, wrestling, or any of the opportunity sports sports or sports activities you are taking a lump on the top.. This does now not even point out what they call sub concussive trauma. That is all the instances you get stung real accurate, however preserve to spar or train as it is not sufficient to prevent you. The extra I discover about head trauma from combative sports activities sports, it turns into a bigger and large element in things like Pugilistic dementia. You can see this in action certainly with the resource of looking at interviews with boxers which have been in the sport for awhile. Look at interviews at the begin in their profession after which on the give up in their careers. You may be capable of see a marked distinction in quite a few of them.

Unless you're the following Floyd Mayweather or Anderson Silva, allow's speak approximately headgear. I actually have more than one diverse types, however maximum are quite sizeable. Headgear is a high-quality issue to have to your gymnasium bag. I absolutely propose having a wonderful set as a manner to protect you. Headgear will no longer save you head trauma best lessen it. But taking a touch masses a whole lot less must add up in a massive manner while you're sixty or seventy. So don't circulate the cheap path for your headgear. Get some component that allows you to do the job but additionally now not forestall you. I without a doubt have a couple of headgear that covers most of my face. That's amazing, but it additionally cuts my imaginative and prescient almost in half. So now I actually have a nice protected head, but cannot see so I get punched within the head more. That negates the gain of have an outstanding included head. What I'm pronouncing fantastic safety with suitable visibility. Please do not use TKD headgear for boxing. It will not protect you nicely. Now I love using TKD headgear for smooth sparring on the ground. It is not so bulky that you can not grapple in it, and it but will guard you from moderate sparring. Also simply due to the reality the fitness center or university you go to has headgear, purchase your very very personal. That manner you realise in which it has been. How antique it's miles, and if it is been wiped smooth well. Plus sporting headgear that has who's aware about how a good deal sweat and blood in is without a doubt gross.

Another vital part of safety, beside your gloves are your hand wraps. These just like most of the machine on this listing are available many patterns. They are available in the entire problem from the same antique hand wrap, at hand wrap gloves, and even the greater expert fashion gauze. You do not have to spend allot of cash available wraps. A couple of first rate hand wraps may be picked up for five-10 bucks. The next detail you want to do is discover ways to wrap them yourself. With a hard and fast of reusable handwraps the coolest element is you can exercise over and over. There are a few notable movies on YouTube that might train you or have a educate train you. Any respectable MMA or putting train can be capable of educate you the way to wrap your hands and need with a view to wrap them until you are proficient at it. The idea at the back of handwrapping is that via wrapping your fingers you're taking the slack out of the bones of the hand. In essence you eliminate a number of the play to your joints, reducing motion of your hand. By doing this you decrease the possibility of injuring your hand at the identical time as you slam it right right right into a bag or each exclusive individual. No one ever hits a intention a one hundred% a 100% of the time. But you can in fact undergo a whole lot much less hand accidents with them properly wrapped. Even for MMA it's miles a exquisite concept to wrap your fingers each time you do any kind of putting. Just think each time you combat your palms may be wrapped, so better get used to it in education. I would possibly have my boxing teach clearly wrap my hands with gauze and tape if I knew we had been going to do a hard sparring consultation with masses of rounds. This way I modified into used to the hand wrap and my hands being wrapped. Just don't forget having your arms wrapped might not cause them to invulnerable. You can however harm them while wrapped but it does provide you with a chunk insurance from damage.

Next is the Mouthpiece. I can't permit you to recognise what number of guys I absolutely have seen that have been round MMA for awhile and though do now not have a mouthpiece that fits. This is one of the most critical things to guard your self from getting KO'd, moreover retaining your very personal enamel. What safety do you have had been given on the identical time because the number one time you open your mouth, your mouthpiece drops on the floor? Not a whole heck of masses. Fitting a mouthpiece properly is not neuroscience, however when you have in no way been confirmed a way to do it, it can be tough to get one to match nicely.

First permit's speak about the types of mouthpieces available. Single ones, double ones, boil and chunk, chemical molded, and professionally molded, are all quite not unusual mouthpieces. Let's take the unmarried mouth piece first. This is the most inexpensive and simplest kind. The boil and chew being the greater commonplace of all of the kinds. I'll get to the high-quality in a minute. These come as cheap as a dollar and up.

The chemical molded ones are to be had in a piece package you combo up and use a dental tray mouthpiece to healthful it. You chunk down and the chemical aggregate hardens and growth straight away mouthpiece. I've in no way used this form of personally, however have heard some of the boxers in my health club bitch about them. I assume it would simply because of the truth they are saying that stuff is nasty tasting.

The subsequent up is a professionally molded mouthpiece. Now going to the dentist is proper enough for a mouthpiece, but there are agencies specializing in now not whatever however mouthpieces for combat sports. Honestly you'll pay certainly little greater but you could get a few component that allows you to guard your tooth. I'm form of attached to mine.

Ok allow's communicate approximately double mouthpieces. My opinion is to throw them inside the trash. In the closing fifteen years I absolutely have in no manner visible one healthy correctly. They all suck badly. They fall out. They don't mold right. They are just now not great mouthpieces for fight sports activities sports sports.

Chapter 7: How to suit a mouthpiece

We are speakme about the incredible antique boil and chunk mouthpiece. I presently have two mouthpieces I keep in my fitness center bag. One is a $1.Ninety seven Franklin mouthpiece. This is by a ways the quality mouthpiece I definitely have ever owned. It is a single boil and bite mouthpiece, but it has some factor I haven't decided in each other. It has raised sections on the lowest of it that allows your jaw to unfold most effective a bit wider apart. It fits remarkable and is more comfortable than each different one I've had. The one-of-a-kind is a $10 surprise medical physician. It isn't as comfortable due to the fact the Franklin however nevertheless a top notch mouthpiece. My issue is you do now not need to spend a ton of cash for a remarkable mouthpiece as lengthy because it suits well.

Now in case you are a professional fighter, pass get a expert mouthpiece. Ok becoming a boil and chew single mouthpiece. First you need to warm temperature it up. I use the microwave. This is an appropriate most available manner. Make awesome that it is right and warm. This is high-quality essential. That mouthpiece desires to be warm. When you boom it out of the cup or bowl it want to nearly melt. I usually throw mine in a cup of cold water for one to 2 seconds, then proper into my mouth. Here is the subsequent most essential hassle. You have to suck at the mouthpiece. This almost vacuum seals it for your enamel. Another nicely trick is to push it up spherical your gums and onto your teeth. Make high-quality to suck. You cannot consider the distinction on the manner to make in the way it suits. After it's far been in your mouth for a minute or so, allow's test the healthful. If it falls from your mouth at the same time as you open it or strive to speak, stick it lower returned inside the microwave and attempt over again. Next do you need to acquire up and pull it out or push it out together with your tongue? If you do, you have got a terrific becoming mouthpiece if you want to guard your grill. I understand mine has stored my tooth a few times. A punch might likely sneak in, proper on the enamel or perhaps an accidental head butt. A pinnacle turning into mouthpiece will save you a set.

Ok we should communicate about circle of relatives protection. Family jewel protection. Athletic cups to be extra particular. To compete you're required to have one. Just like a mouthpiece you need a cup that is going to in form properly and defend you thoroughly. I now not regularly put on one once I'm in beauty, but in reality ought to have used one a time or .

Just like all of the different device, there are numerous types of cups out there. There are the everyday three greenback baseball cups after which all the manner up to the Muay Thai steel cup. The Muay Thai style steel cup is through using a ways the amazing safety, but occasionally may be difficult to get an extraordinary match. I myself pick a respectable marvel medical doctor type cup with the flexible facets in order that they do not lessen into my thighs, just like the metallic cup can. As my partner says I'm constructed like a gorilla. You want one which fits. Lose the ego and get one this is cushty and will guard you. I had been training and competing for a long term, so I simply have taken some nasty images within the southern vicinity. I even have had a couple of testicular torsions from the ones pix.

Now if you don't know what this is here's the short anatomy lesson. It is even as the testicles twist together by means of the twine retaining them. It is outstanding painful. I did no longer think masses about this because it had generally went away with some days rest and some Advil. But the closing time it did no longer go away. I had a testicular torsion multiple years ago which did not unwrap itself. I needed to be prepped for emergency surgical treatment after in step with week of herbal hell. They took considered one among testicles and had been able to maintain the alternative. Two weeks later I advanced an automobile immune sickness that took me from expert athlete to a 90 one year antique man. For the following six months I could nearly cry every time I had to stroll up or down a flight of stairs. Luckily after approximately a twelve months and a half of of going to clinical docs and no longer getting any solutions I in the long run located some answers from of all places, an OB/GYN. She modified right into a hormone expert and have become able to positioned me again on a healthful route. I am however no longer again to the location I changed into in advance than all of this however I am truly better than I turn out to be. The ethical of this story is, placed on the cup. It is a relative much less costly piece of device that is probably capable of save you a ton of ache and grief.

Make certain to also get a extremely good fitting jock strap or some form of modular device to hold the cup in location. It received't do you plenty nicely if it acquired't live in which it is supposed to. I apprehend there are a few groups on hand that make a compression short with an equal cup. This is a extremely good investment as a fighter. Now for all the lady opponents available they do make some variations for girls, however as a long way as I recognise they may be now not required in opposition. But after further dialogue with my spouse, getting kicked inside the woman elements does no longer enjoy real appropriate. So girls it could no longer be a awful investment to your training.

Another exceptional piece of device to have is a couple of shin guards. I do propose getting the Muay Thai fashion shin guards. I recognize there are the cloth padded ones available very reasonably-priced, but please get some first rate Thai fashion shin guards. This is protection on your shins however extra importantly it's far protection to your sparring partners. You will understand if you have ever been kicked thru a naked shin the pain that it could inflict. It truly hurts. If you don't take transport of as actual with me allow honestly one in all your friends come up with a mild roundhouse to the outdoor of your thigh. Now while you could stand and use your leg all over again we're able to preserve. Me in my view in case you aren't sporting shin guards I will no longer spar with you the usage of kicks. I have been silly inside the past and have injured my feet, my shins, and my knees. Just recollect it, you're in a pleasing tough sparring consultation, you're getting a chunk worn-out. You drop your palms for a 2d and increase shin to move. See glove reference above. Shots to the pinnacle motive brain damage climate it's miles a kick or a punch. Now with shin guards and headgear on, the blow may additionally need to had been masses certainly considered one of a kind. It possibly may additionally have although harm however it may be the distinction among persevering with your education that night time or sitting down on the point of the mat cause you currently see 3 of the whole lot.

You don't need to have all the incredible tool to train MMA, but at least spend the cash to get extremely good gadget. I realise one of the things I truely have run into over time is that warring parties as a group are normally pretty broke. But in case you are truly important about schooling it does take cash. This is probably a reoccurring component. It takes coins for a educate or commands, it takes coins for tool, it takes coins to journey and it takes cash to food regimen successfully. There is a ton of agencies now promoting combat sports activities sports sports system. Even Wal-Mart sells MMA tool.

The subsequent piece is a should in case you are going to do jiu jitsu, a gi. This is greater than a uniform. It is a tool, a chunk of device a good manner to hone your abilities to a razors issue. My first actual experience with the gi become once I took

Hapkido for some years. This emerge as the number one time the gi or uniform I wore changed into used as a weapon, a cope with, or a device. If you come back from a wrestling historical past like I do the gi is set as one-of-a-type because it receives. It is absolutely distant places. But at the same time as you start to get the cling of it opens up dimensions to the grappling activity that you didn't understand wherein there. I didn't have pretty a few admire for the gi till my instructor threw me then choked me with it approximately 5 times in a row. Then it took me a few years after that to return lower decrease lower back to it.

I recognize you are questioning why grappling in a gi might make me higher at MMA. Let's start with method. Almost all grappling technique can be tailor-made to gi or no gi. Grappling within the gi will make you greater technical. I stated this changed into BS on the start. I realize now why I idea this. I have emerge as adapting nogi jiu jitsu and wrestling to gi jiu jitsu. That meant I modified into skipping probably thirds of every approach. You can get away with a lot extra at the same time as your opponent isn't capable of take maintain of you. The gi is sort of a large manage. It can slow the entirety all the manner down to the same of WW1 trench war. Here is the first detail as a way to raise your game. Grips. Whether it is getting your grips or breaking your opponents grips. The act of having to be cognizant of in that you placed your arms and wherein your opponent locations his is now a very important detail. Jimmy Pedro, Olympian and Olympic train summed it up awesome," He who wins the grips wins the combat." The gi can be the notable equalizer of duration and electricity. It slows the pace at times, and permits you to manipulate a much larger opponent. It is lots greater of a weapon than I had ever believed. In hapkido we used the gi, however it modified into in a rudimentary manner in assessment to Brazilian jiu jitsu. Hapkido became one of the first hybrid arts combining multi disciplines into one. When you try this it is difficult to specialize the art. Brazilian jiu jitsu has had a hundred years of refining the grappling art inside the gi. I went from information a few chokes with the gi to reading over a dozen nearly right now, with in all likelihood masses greater.

Let's talk approximately gis. There are honestly loads of numerous sorts, patterns, and shades to pick out from. The first detail you want to do is discover whether or not or now not the gym you are attending has any policies on sorts or sun sun shades of gis which can be accredited. I've been to a few schools that it modified into obligatory that the gi be white or blue with best the colleges patches. Then a few I've been to permit any shade or style of jiu jitsu gi. My personal university I allow any color so long as it's far smooth and in well order. I come from a place in which tae kwon do may be very well-known so guys will are available in and ask if they may positioned on their antique TKD uniforms. This is not a large trouble with me, however I normally tell them they will want to buy a bjj gi earlier than lengthy. Just because the thin gi will now not stand up to the beating your gi will take at some stage in magnificence. I even have six gis I rotate carrying. I actually have a couple which can be cheaper than the others, however I actually have a pair that I paid hundreds extra cash for.

Gis are like most property you pay for pleasant and you pay for the decision. What I endorse to most men is buy one via the school that you are at on your first gi. This suggests a dedication on your university and it might be a notable enough gi. I use Century Martial Arts for my student gis. I attempt to get them to my university college students as cheap as possible. They make a superb gi for an inexpensive rate. Remember men it does no longer should be a particular bjj gi. It may be a judo or robust shade hapkido gi also. These kinds are almost same to bjj gis. I additionally recommend while men can get a second gi and rotate them. This will in reality expand the life of your gis. I understand a variety of my men take lots of pride in their gis. I will talk about cleansing and maintaining your gis in a later bankruptcy.

The next piece of device is what is called a rash defend. This is the tight stretchy ready shirt which you see worn below the gi or at the same time as someone is doing a nogi grappling healthy. The rash guard originated with surf culture and changed into tailor-made to jiu jitsu. The rash protect is super at minimizing the chaffing you get collectively along with your gi or from the mat. Plus who desires to roll round with some sweaty dude without a shirt on. Personally I revel in more mobile even as carrying one opposed to carrying a t-blouse below my gi, sparring, or at the same time as rolling. With a t-blouse it is truly a few different layer of clothing to gradual me down. But the rash guard will simply reduce down on surely what the decision implies. It guards from rash associated with rolling in a gi or on the mat. It is likewise being finished in maximum nogi grappling tournaments. It cuts down on getting your hand caught in a t-shirt within the middle of a competition. Plus all once more who desires to rub on a few sweaty stranger if you do now not need to.

Here is every other piece of machine that isn't 100% crucial, however does make grappling or MMA a piece higher, and that is the MMA quick or board shorts. I can not say they'll make your recreation any higher but they're generally masses extra long lasting than ordinary exercising or gym shorts. The MMA short has got here an extended manner inside the last few years. They are designed to be the least resistive as feasible. They lead them to in every colour and masses of styles. There are some made to be microbial and bacterial resistant. They cause them to out of rip forestall fabric made to reason them to more long lasting. Just like the any of the device you get what you pay for. Like I said earlier than it isn't always clearly critical to have and if it comes all the manner proper right down to getting your gadget or getting the present day-day cool combat shorts, get your machine. I understand it's far a part of the MMA and grappling life-style to have notable combat shorts, but prioritize what you need. We will speak approximately the lifestyle in a later chapter and the way it has affected the sports activities and those who educate them. Remember combat shorts are a few different present from the Brazilian surf way of life. Fight shorts are in reality fancy board shorts. So if you want some in a pinch hit nearby save for some board shorts. Don't forget about to attempt not get people with wallet however if you do no zippers please. You can usually positioned a piece of Velcro to close up the pockets.

So we have protected most of the simple device you want for mixed martial arts or for Brazilian jiu jitsu. Lets recap the fundamentals. The first for each undertaking is the mats. If you are doing truely Jiu Jitsu or grappling you then are in business agency so to talk. If you have a

MMA fitness center you can need at least a heavy bag. That is as primary because it receives in your place. If you don't take delivery of as true with me simply take a look at out had been the Gracies began training jiu jitsu out of in California, a storage. We have run thru the basics of your private device that you'll be wanting additionally. There may be a tick list at the surrender of this e-book you could use to look if you have left out some thing.

Here are a few more portions of system that aren't a extremely good critical, however I idea I might throw it in right right here. The first is a grappling dummy. There are numerous types and patterns. Some of the most clean patterns are what I first skilled in high university wrestling. It is a sure throwing dummy. It is normally about 5 foot tall, someplace among 70-80 kilos and has two immediately hands sticking out of it. This is terrific for what its name implies, throwing. It isn't in reality first rate for grappling or takedowns. It commonly doesn't have legs. These dummies usually run a couple hundred greenbacks. Not actual rate inexperienced besides you actually need to art work on the few wrestling or judo throws you may do with it. The next dummy is a step up from this however pretty an awful lot the same except that it has legs. These are better for additonal conventional takedowns, however nonetheless not the great for grappling. The stiff arms and legs will can help you paintings some submissions however no longer too many. These dummies are a bit greater highly-priced than the last. The subsequent one is sincerely greater of what we'd name a grappling dummy. The big aspect that separates this is the capability to transport and pose the arms and legs. If you preferred to work on a few detail from kimuras, armbars, heel hooks or chokes.

You may even paintings in defend, for passing or sweeps. These dummies are quite a bit greater luxurious than the previous, however they allow you to attain this a superb deal greater. They assist you to drill pretty a few strategies for your private. If you need examples of drills you may do in truth check YouTube or simply lookup dummy schooling DVDs. Know those dummies are costly so I wouldn't use them for putting. That is what you've got got got your heavy bag for. Also they do make a few setting dummies best for ground paintings. I myself should never locate the cash for this type of fancy grappling dummies so started out out searching out thoughts to make my non-public. I honestly have to say there are a collection of a manner to movies on making your very very own dummy. This is what I did. I without a doubt have to mention I spent approximately $30 dollars and a few hours and now I without a doubt have a high-quality schooling companion who by no means complains. So test out YouTube and strive making your personal. I understand this is not an important piece of tool however it's far sincerely a laugh to have and to scare the crap out of your spouse with via leaving it in sudden places.

The next is get right of entry to to statistics. Whether the statistics comes from a e-book, a DVD, or the net, it's far generally right to start constructing a library of information. There is lots records obtainable nowadays it is hard to type via all of it. There is right, lousy, and certainly simple terrible info available. We will cover the way to use the ones as a getting to know device later.

It is usually right to complement your statistics from wonderful sources. The super manner of direction is to have a informed educate, but from time to time this is not the manner it virtually works out. You could be conscious that positive moves or holds are quite normal while you check out DVDs, books, or YouTube. My advice is test out reviews, ask round, and satisfactory get your facts from in a position assets. MMA champions and jiu jitsu champions are constantly a outstanding location to begin. Then recollect to strive the men that coached those champions, in particular in case you are going to drop the cash for a ebook or DVD. Ask your educate or instructor. They can will let you understand some extremely good property.

Now allow's communicate about the most controversial of the 3 mediums, YouTube. Here is one of the splendid instances to stick to my earlier advice. Look for champions or coaches of champions. These guys are generally your brilliant desire for facts for strategies, weight manipulate, and cardio/power education. Granted there are men to be had that aren't champions and also have unique educational motion pictures, however be cautious watch loads of movement images, take notes and examine. Most primary strategies pretty much every person can train, it's only some educate it higher than others. This is every other problem count I will take a look at on this ebook, credibility. Choose credible instructors. Here is a exquisite supply away. If the video is filmed in someone's basement and seems like it might be part of snuff movie, find each different video. There also are some tremendous web sites which are now setting collectively breakdowns of champion fighters mainly in the BJJ network. Check out considered certainly one of my favorites Bishopbjj.Com's breakdown of champion BJJ opponents.

Here is one brief piece of gadget you want to have if you are going to compete. It does not recollect if it's far MMA, wrestling, nogi grappling, or jiu jitsu. You need a digital scale. Let me be a bit clearer a DIGITAL SCALE. Being a MMA promoter while you get men pass over an agreed upon weight for a fight or grappling in shape. It is one of the maximum worrying things within the international. You get the ones men who are actually tremendous amazed that they disregarded their weight. I continuously ask what did you weigh for your scale and what shape of scale became it? Most of the time it's far on the cheap old spring kind relaxation room scales. These are a number of the maximum faulty scales stated to guy. I even get guys who don't weigh themselves in any respect, however the ones are commonly 130lbs guys who're preventing 155lbs and say I've been consuming looking for to place on some weight.

Anyway if you are going to compete in any recreation that calls on the way to make a tremendous weight, please buy a digital scale. It does not have to be a $500 medical physician's scale, however don't buy the $5.Ninety nine approach each. You can get a decent digital scale for round $20 dollars. As a promoter I beg you to do this. It will save you a few heartache in case you are in reality slicing weight to make a weight elegance. If you grow to be a seasoned MMA fighter it will make a distinction on you paycheck. Ok, non-public tool, you can want the following. Some of it you can want greater than others. The first portions of tool are the gloves. You will want boxing and MMA gloves. Remember there are hundreds of these gloves out inside the interwebs. Just do some research on brands and one of a kind styles. You are awesome to find out a few which may be appropriate for you. The subsequent on the listing is headgear.

Get a few proper headgear with appropriate visibility. Get a few thing on the manner to guard your gourd. Then we referred to mouthpieces. Single over double whenever. It does no longer need to be costly, but it does want to healthful nicely. Then we cited cups. This is insurance for destiny fitness and legacy. A right turning into cup is critical to defensive the circle of relatives jewels. Don't get the cup you had even as you played little league baseball. Get a muay thai metallic cup. They closing all the time and could guard you. Then we come to shin guards. Muay thai equipment is the incredible manner to go together with this one yet again. Don't buy tae kwon do shin guards. They do not guard you the manner you want to be blanketed. You and your partner will be glad which you spend a touch extra and get Muay Thai fashion. We come to the gis. Remember judo or jiu jitsu student gis are flawlessly fine to apply. Then whilst you could discover the cash for it get you one which's all patched up, with a constructed in rash shield and has rip prevent cloth. Rashguards can be surely bjj rashguards, surf fashion rash guards, or only a easy as an below armor style compression shirt. Fight shorts or grappling shorts, are a need to for MMA or nogi grappling. Here is the name of the game to combat shorts, they are some different thing added from surf life-style. They are board shorts. Thank the Brazilians over again for this addition. The remaining at the list is the grappling dummy. If you have got were given the cash to drop for one of the fancy ones incredible, however if you are on a fee range like me, check out YouTube for incredible methods to make your own reasonably-priced. I love mine. It is to be had in accessible for max top drills and even some backside drills. The very last piece is DVDs, books, and the internet.

Find credible resources for you records. It typically facilitates to keep mastering. Just do not go to elegance with a few wacky method you found on YouTube and count on it to trump the whole thing else. I'll make this one short. Buy a virtual scale. I'm sure I forgot some thing, however this listing covers most of the highlights of essential device you may need for MMA, grappling, or jiu jitsu.

Chapter 8: MMA History

Mixed Martial Arts is one of the oldest prepared sports activities sports sports referred to to guy. It is also one of the oldest hand handy fight models utilized by militaries anywhere inside the international. The Greeks referred to as it Pankration, and it dates yet again to 600 B.C. It is humorous most traditional martial artists chuckle at mixed martial arts and the manner untraditional it is. That's humorous due to how vintage the requirements of blended martial arts are. Warriors were using the precept of mixed martial arts for thousands of years. It is the principle of slicing away the fats out of a martial arts device and the usage of what works in fight, and now days what works in competition.

Mixed martial arts are using placing and grappling techniques, each standing and at the floor. Mixed martial arts bouts have taken region all over the global during the last hundred years in Europe, Japan, South America, and the us. They have simplest really come into the limelight during the last two decades. This end up with the assist of the mythical Gracie Family from Brazil. The Gracie own family spawned the UFC and brought NHB occasions all through the USA and South America. The first UFC premiered in 1993 and with a few growing pains has grown proper proper into a international phenomenon. It commenced as what turn out to be known as a No holds barred competition. It changed into a contest of style in opposition to fashion, with restrained policies and no cut-off dates. The handiest pointers in the first contests were, no biting, no eye gouging, and no fish hooking. Everything else emerge as jail. Royce Gracie dominated the early competitions with Brazilian jiu jitsu, some difficulty that had not frequently been seen outside of his local Brazil. This might be very important considering Royce become an unassuming almost thin 180lb youngster on the time.

The game persevered to conform with the addition of extra rules, ultimate dates, and gloves. The style instead of fashion problem remember changed into quick changed thru the number one generation of proper contemporary-day blended martial artists. They started out schooling inside the entirety from boxing, kickboxing, wrestling, judo, and of path Brazilian Jiu Jitsu. The athletes have turn out to be international class technicians of many patterns and techniques. The athletes have become large, faster, and stronger. The strategies of MMA have emerge as so powerful it has drawn the eye of a number of the fine militaries inside the world, together with the usa Military. The US Military Combative programs are nearly solely drawn from the techniques of cutting-edge blended martial arts. The US Military even has their non-public Combative tournaments to test the skills of the soldiers. This is most effective a short synopsis on the statistics of MMA, but with like numerous martial arts mastering is a in no way completing adventure. Go test out the records of MMA and the UFC.

MMA Schools

Ok turning into a member of a MMA gymnasium may be actually fantastic revel in, wherein you may forge a state-of-the-art you within the crucible of combat or it can be a miserable enjoy that you could in no way ever want to move back again to yet again. The traditional martial arts college is often a lot greater hooked up and formal than most MMA schools or perhaps Brazilian Jiu Jitsu faculties. Everyone is predicted to bow and answer positive sir to all questions in a noisy projecting voice. MMA schools tend to be the polar opposite of conventional martial arts faculties. You can almost say MMA schools are the darkish aspect of martial arts. Mixed martial arts schools have a tendency to be masses greater bodily than traditional martial arts schools. Yes, you usually have a few contact at some point of conventional martial arts, however with MMA you may have a whole lot of bodily touch, besides you are taking a cagefighting fitness beauty. I will come up with some scoop on those instructions a touch later furthermore. Most MMA instructors are commonly masses more laid once more than your ultra-modern traditional martial arts trainer. You do not get the equal vibe you get in a conventional martial arts elegance. I've been lucky even if I actually have studied traditional martial arts my teachers had been more unconventional and it did now not revel in like I modified into in a inflexible conventional martial arts splendor. One of the belongings you need to do in advance than going to a MMA university is decide how an lousy lot contact you're inclined to take. One of the subjects I offer my college students is the capability to determine out of stay sparring. This eases pretty a few anxiety, however then every so often that nasty ego rears its head and they do it except. I try and sit down down and communicate with every scholar and get their expectations of what they need out of class. I will speak the ego in a later monetary disaster.

Choosing a MMA School

Now in case you are from a city like mine there had been no MMA faculties. Even now there are not any MMA schools, except for mine. I would love to count on it's far due to the fact I am such an wonderful trainer that I ran each person out of commercial business enterprise. Unfortunately I suppose it is without a doubt the size of the town I stay in. You additionally thing in the paintings it takes to take part in MMA and the bodily contact. It makes MMA a totally fringe martial artwork. Most people would possibly as an opportunity take a seat down at home and watch it on TV than get in the health club and established thirty hours of labor every week on the MMA fitness center. I even have to inform you most guys do not live with MMA. The longest I've had any scholar changed into for four years. Most closing to a few months. This is not because I am so super tough at the guys. It is simply that MMA is tremendous tough, especially in case you need to compete. That is each distinct massive problem you need to determine in advance than going to class.

Do you need to compete or just get in form. So permit's say your town does have more than one MMA college. It's time to choose. First thing you need to do is go to the faculties. Here is in which you acquire your intel. You need to discover as an awful lot about the colleges as you can. You need to discover one on the manner to fit you, and moreover one which you'll in form in to as nicely.

We will begin at the pinnacle, instructors. Find out if it's far one trainer or multiple teachers. You need to recognize why the teachers are certified to teach the schooling you need to take. A lot of colleges offer multiple commands like putting, wrestling, Brazilian jiu jitsu, and sparring instructions. Find out the credentials for each trainer. Don't run out if the trainer isn't a international champion, and do not anticipate if he's that he is probably a super teach. The trainer's credentials are just a place to begin whilst choosing a university. If you're searching for to come to be a fighter ask if the college has a fight team. Ask in the event that they have any pro combatants. Ask inside the occasion that they have amateur combatants competing regionally. If the school has men which can be competing specially if they have seasoned opponents competing, as a manner to inform you they as a minimum have in vicinity a number of the subjects you can want to grow to be a fighter. Ask if the university is a part of an association. This is extra famous with Brazilian jiu jitsu and greater traditional martial arts than it's far with MMA, but there are a few available. My MMA university have become a part of the Miletich Fighting Systems school back a few years within the beyond. This became a outstanding employer, however we have been without a doubt no longer able to preserve the affiliation going. This did not make my university that a wonderful deal higher than others it simply gave us more possibilities to transport and teach places and to make connections. So virtually ask approximately the affiliation. It surely creates extra opportunities.

Next you could want to take a excursion of the school. There are some property you need to look for. The first just like we said at the beginning is a mat area. It is ninety nine.9%, sincerely vital that the university have a mat region. Now it does now not should be 8000 square feet, however it does need to thoroughly accommodate all the university students in elegance. There is not anything worse than having to sit down at the facet of the mat because of the fact there isn't room to paintings in class. Do they have got a cage, ring, or cage wall of some type. Just like we talked about earlier, you want to have some manner to artwork on the cage or simulate walking on the cage. I without a doubt have watched guys from faculties that did not have this, and you could see the hole in their game. This is at the amateur diploma. I could not hold in mind a seasoned fighter no longer gaining access to this a part of MMA education.

Ok the subsequent large aspect is instructions and class availability. Most MMA schools may additionally moreover have training three to five times a week. Please don't routinely think if a university does not provide commands seven days every week it is a waste of time. Three is type of the minimum of sophistication days that can be furnished and it is virtually worth becoming a member of. Classes need to be at least an hour lengthy depending what they'll be and some also can need to be longer. You will need at the least class types, putting and grappling.

Some schools will offer hundreds greater instructions, however the ones are the bare minimal if you want to be an MMA fighter.

Class Breakdown

Grappling Class

This class wants to educate you, the entirety from standup wrestling, takedowns, and ground paintings, along side submissions and submission defenses. These should all be classes via themselves, but you need to get all of those gadgets for a grappling beauty to advantage you. Expect touch from a grappling beauty. This is an absolute want to in case you are going to be taking an MMA elegance. Now you have to ask if you have the choice to take a seat down out of any sparring or rolling that you don't sense comfortable with. Any reasonable instructor will answer sure of direction. If an trainer calls for you to be in every sparring or rolling consultation you must probably query if that university is an area you need to be. This generally reminds of women who could likely come to beauty, and ask do I ought to roll spherical with sweaty men. Well sure to a point. You need to perform a bit degree of grappling to be in a grappling elegance. So for all of the girls on hand in case you are inquisitive about an MMA or grappling elegance, just be ready to roll with guys in some unspecified time within the destiny in elegance. If you take this beauty for self protection competencies, you'll in truth want to roll with the guys in beauty.

You don't clearly pay attention ladies being mugged or attacked by using manner of various women.

So ensure the splendor teaches the 3 stuff you need in a grappling beauty.

Standup wrestling, takedowns, and ground work.

Also make sure to ask if sitting out of sparring or rolling is Ok?

Striking Class

A placing magnificence might be in truely considered one of patterns. Boxing or kickboxing. This is a massive stroke for hanging, but we are speakme about MMA. Boxing is a reasonably easy transition to teach for MMA. Boxing for MMA will need to be tweaked in apprehend to all the other components of MMA. Two of these elements being takedowns and kick defense. The takedown part of this ought to be protected to your grappling class, but have to moreover be covered at the least in element on your placing class. The subsequent detail is kicks. If you're in a herbal boxing elegance, this could probable now not be covered. If the college does not provide a few form of kickboxing you'll need to pursue some education on at least kick protection. I virtually have visible some top notch combatants in no way throw a kick, however you may wager they certain apprehend a way to protect them.

Kickboxing is the excellent of every worlds. I experience the satisfactory kickboxing style for MMA is Muay Thai kickboxing. I recognise there are one of a kind kinds of martial arts that use kicks, like Tae Kwon Do and Karate. I even have visible seasoned warring parties use those patterns and be very a hit with them. One of Muay Thai's crucial advantages is the simplicity of the techniques to study. I virtually have seen guys select up the essential kicks and knees with as low as some weeks schooling. Not to mention Muay Thai fashion elbows are some of the most dangerous guns inside the putting arsenal. You will also be learning the simple defenses inside the route of kicks and elbows.

Once you've got seen what style of setting elegance you will also need to invite if the sparring is non-obligatory or no longer. If you are in reality an enthusiast who isn't always looking for to combat, not sparring is Ok. If you're a fighter, you need to spar. It's shape of like fight membership. If it's your first night time time at fight club, you need to combat. We will cowl sparring a piece later. Also if you are doing MMA or putting for self protection you will need to spar furthermore. Remember this at the same time as you are looking at instructions.

We protected the 2 easy instructions colleges have to provide for primary MMA. Here are some training wonderful schools provide except the essential MMA commands.

Chapter 9: Sparring Class

Some colleges offer a night time particularly for sparring. If you are a fighter that may be a should to attend. This is often a magnificence for university college students who want to beautify their sensible martial arts talents or who want to fight. If you suggest on attending a class like this, count on the occasional bloody nose or wrenched arm. This is wherein method meets exercise in a managed environment. We will communicate the etiquette worried in sparring a chunk later additionally.

Conditioning or Cardio Cagefighting Class

This is simply what it says, a category so that it will paintings your conditioning. Most conditioning or aerobic instructions will do fight unique kind drills. A lot of these instructions are advertised as train like a fighter type instructions. This a splendid beauty to go to if you want to be in form like a fighter without the drawbacks of going to a category in that you are getting punched within the face.

Brazilian Jiu Jitsu Class

This is regularly furnished at many large or extra numerous gyms. Jiu Jitsu is a gi grappling art work, began out via the Gracie family in Brazil. This might be the most well-known grappling art work within the worldwide, besides wrestling. You don't ought to do gi jiu jitsu to do MMA, but it does help together with your grappling sport or floor abilties.

We protected the crucial varieties of schooling. Don't overlook at a few huge schools those training also can also be broke up further into novices and advanced university college students. The subsequent trouble whilst selecting a college, does the education you need to wait, coordinate with the nights you're available to attend training. That is a big locating out element for selecting a university. Here is the large one which receives lots of people. PRICE$$$. The fee may be very important because of the truth, you need rate to your dollar. You don't need to move straight away to the most inexpensive faculty you may discover. And vice versa, virtually due to the truth a faculty is the most high-priced college does now not mean it's far the great faculty. This is one the number one reasons I am putting all this down on paper is to help with the tough selections. Definitely preserve round. I've have given you some actual particular subjects to begin looking for in an MMA college. The belongings you need to search for are, what does the charge embody: all of the schooling, some of the classes, or one class. Do they offer a one charge consists of all? Is there a sign on price? If so do you get some thing together with your be part of up rate, like t-blouse or shorts? Are the month-to-month dues installation on a bank with draw device or do you truly make payments on the college each month. Some schools offer reductions in case you use the financial institution with draw gadget, but endure in thoughts, similarly they'll price you the the rest of your agreement in case you pick out out early or they will price you for an extra month cancelation price. These are all questions you need to invite, in advance than signing any contracts. Always ask if you could attempt some training out earlier than signing up. This is every other deal breaker, if a college obtained't at the least let you attempt a category or it isn't well worth attending.

The closing factor approximately deciding on a MMA faculty is rating. This is a few element very arguable within the MMA global. Mixed martial arts are the conglomeration of many martial arts. So how does one get a rank in a few issue this is fabricated from so many special martial arts. This is an easy one. Someone simply has to begin the rating gadget and a curriculum. Ranking structures are in particular a manner for a student to peer accomplishment alongside a certain route. MMA is not so specific from the beginnings of many special martial arts. It is fight examined and sensitive to a more natural version of what works. So why now not rank students. The biggest fighters usually come from the traditional guys. From my experience the conventional men usually don't apprehend MMA an entire lot first of all. So that could be a suitable question to ask about the school. Does the college rank in MMA? A lot of the ranking I even have seen in MMA is mostly a hybrid shape of a conventional martial paintings. So if you don't take transport of as proper with in MMA belt score you may commonly ask Matt Hughes, former UFC Welterweight champion and black belt beneath Pat Miletich's Miletich Fighting Systems. Or the guys from Greg Jackson's Martial Arts

You want to simply take all of these items under attention even as selecting your college. I preference a number of those questions help you at the same time as you are making your choice. Also in no manner allow all of us decide for you. I apprehend if perhaps you get a few loose months education as a present. These paragraphs above have to give you an wonderful begin for choosing a university. Remember it is extremely tough to discover a university that meets all the standards, however use your fantastic judgment, and ask questions. If you can, truely speak to the human beings at the university. Talk to the instructor, in case you experience right approximately the situation join up and begin down the street to being a blended martial artist, perhaps even the subsequent champ of the sector.

A Typical Mixed Martial Arts Class

We have noted some of the varieties of commands you can assume to peer at a blended martial arts college. Now allow's speak about what you could expect on the instructions themselves. Most combined martial arts schooling have a study a few form of this clean device. You can also have a few sort of warmth-up, determined by way of method, a few shape of sparring, and generally surrender with a aerobic exercise of some type. This system is used at some of the most essential faculties all the way all the manner all the manner down to the smallest. This is the layout that I use for most of the instructions I train.

Warm-america of americaare generally ten minutes to 15 mins long. I wanted everyone to have as a minimum a light sweat going into the technique part of the magnificence. The technique element is usually the red meat of the splendor. Depending at the beauty, the method factor modified into commonly approximately forty-five mins to an hour. Here is some other tip I found out along the way for teaching college students. Never teach more than 3 strategies and if you could, link the three techniques. It makes it easier to analyze and to maintain. Retention of method, as a student is wonderful crucial, and as an instructor being able to teach so your college college students are able to hold facts is simply as vital.

The next element is the sparring. I typically had the men do as a minimum some form of sparring. Really seeking to get the guys to position into impact the things they truely discovered in elegance. Ultimately, you want your university college students so you can carry out strategies on an opponent at almost entire tempo or at complete tempo. The closing thing of sophistication may additionally need to extra often than no longer include a few type of aerobic exercising. This turn out to be commonly best about ten mins, but it have come to be a incredible way to cap off class. The exercise almost always consisted of body weight physical sports activities or particular drills for MMA. This will provide you with some element to count on from maximum combined martial arts or grappling lessons. There are distinct elegance codecs obtainable but maximum will stick fantastically near this sample.

Warm Up

We begin with the superb and cushty up. Most colleges need to have a slight warmth up. Usually this isn't that difficult in case you are in shape the least bit. If you are just turning into a member of the beauty after years of Xbox education, don't be discouraged if you can't make it via the warm up. This isn't a big deal, however you can want to get in which you could. My concept is that if the terrific and relaxed up is providing you with issues, exercising it at home. It generally takes very little region to exercise. You instructor will apprehend you placing forth the try to keep up with the magnificence. Believe me, magnificence will generally run smoother if every person can preserve up. Not to mention you may be beaten if you may't preserve up, however please placed forth the strive. One of the things I cherished approximately being an instructor became when I made an effect on my students. Seeing them emerge as extra physically healthy have come to be honestly this type of adjustments. You is probably surprised how little it takes to end up greater healthful. Fifteen mins of working towards the primary heat u.S. Home will have you getting thru it in beauty right away. What are typically some of the primary warmness ups. You can use this to be organized in case you want to get a jumpstart on elegance.

Here is one which I commonly use for my essential combined martial arts beauty. We begin with shrimping. If you're now pronouncing what the hell does that want to do with martial arts, please absolutely appearance it up on YouTube. This might be one of the most vital talents you could have at the ground. The subsequent one we'd do is a shoulder stroll. It is actually what it says. Lay flat to your again and stroll your shoulders down the mat. Next we'd do what I affectionately name

Lieutenant Dan's. This warmth-up is in which you lay flat in your belly and pull your self across the floor collectively at the side of your arms high-quality, no legs. I recognize this is an antique Forest Gump reference, however if you have to invite. I name this workout Lt. Dan's is because of the fact Lt. Dan doesn't have any legs. I realize cheesy, however it makes me snigger every time I say it in elegance.

Then we would skip directly to the maximum disturbing exercise I have ever had the revel in of doing. It is called a rocking chair. I understand this could be tough to describe the incredible frustration humans have with this workout until you could sincerely enjoy it for your self. I became demonstrated this exercising via taken into consideration one among my head Brazilian Jiu Jitsu teachers. The outstanding Royler Gracie black belt JW Wright. I recognize cheap plug. What you do is lay flat in your lower back. Bring your knees barely up and start a small rocking movement. This is the smooth part of the exercise. Next while persevering with your rocking motion; convey your arms inside the path of the ceiling. Drop your palms for your left as your hips pass to the right. Then through bringing your arms once more to your proper it brings your shoulders over some inches to the right. You just keep repeating the method, moving your manner down the mat sideways. Rocking all the even as you swing your palms one route and hips the opposite. I'm getting aggravated just talking approximately it. But there may be desire. Once this workout clicks and it does for maximum oldsters after a few rounds, it is a tremendous belly workout.

Then we bypass onto beforehand rolling wreck falls. It is a clean judo exercise for movement and balance. Another one you can discover a ton of movement pics showing you the manner to do. Break falling is a high-quality crucial talent to take a look at irrespective of what martial artwork you are taking. After the judo break falls, I typically have the students do some particular forms of animal drills. Like alligator taking walks, undergo crawls, and frog hops. These are also splendid drills for warming up, but moreover running on stability and coordination. The heat up is sort of completed. The subsequent drill I may have the elegance do is what is referred to as an upa. It is a shoulder bridge. Basically you lay flat to your once more with legs bent and ft on the floor. You will then enhance your hips off the ground proper proper into a bridge feature. While your hips are in the air, you may collect one hand up excessive over the possibility shoulder. You are seeking to roll on the opportunity shoulder and speak to the floor as a long way decrease returned as you may. This is a number one wrestling drill. If you look for shoulder bridges on YouTube, you can discover this on there. Typically I could have the magnificence do fifty upas twenty five on each thing. This could probably lead into some essential body weight bodily video games. I even have three which are my bread and butter warmth ups. The first exercise is the pushup. The next exercise may be the sit up straight. The remaining of the three might be a frame weight squat. All of those sports are fifty repetitions as a minimum. When I had fine a class of fighters it come to be a hundred and fifty reps and they had ten minutes to finish all of them. For maximum of the men this modified into now not a trouble. This is the fundamental heat up for maximum of the commands I taught. I could not take into account doing anymore than this warmth up, handiest for time constraint competencies. I in reality have seen some colleges do heat-americathat lasted as plenty as thirty mins. I do expect all of us to get thru the satisfactory and cozy up, however it doesn't want to be the primary time through them.

Technique

The subsequent a part of my training might be approach and drills. I couldn't even recall list all of the strategies that it's miles viable to train. I will will let you know some thing as a manner to help. It is to only train 3 strategies a class. If you teach any extra than which you run the threat of your university university college students no longer being able to hold the records. And in case your trainer does teach more than three techniques in a night time recognition on 3 of these techniques. One of the subjects I typically do as a scholar is write the strategies down as quickly as I get out of class or I get domestic. I genuinely have an app on my mobile phone that is a jiu Jitsu log ebook. I then switch all my hand written scribbles into this log. It is a pleasant little app. It categorizes all of the techniques and drills. But if you need to preserve the things you look at in class, write them down. I even have notebooks and notebooks of techniques I actually have found out over the years. Make superb you placed an define of processes the method works also. Because going again years later and reviewing your scribbles, it could be from time to time tough to decipher what you have got been considering at the time. The app sincerely helps you to add photos or video with the approach furthermore. This is available in accessible. The final beauty I taught we have been filming strategies and putting them on YouTube for the beauty to check. With the Jiu Jitsu Log app I need to load those movement pictures proper at the log and characteristic a visible reference. You can also hyperlink one thousand precise movies from YouTube.

Writing it down is simplest a reminiscence technique, but it is been validated to help together with your retention. It can be used with masses of numerous matters, remembering humans's call is a large one. Just write them down and companion a few detail with it. Just like writing the method down, accomplice the facts of the technique with it. We also do masses of drilling during this time. Drilling is the first-class manner to cement the muscle reminiscence part of analyzing a way. This is a simple reading concept. Drill the approach till you no longer need to bear in mind the technique. This is an crucial capacity you want to examine whether you are doing martial arts for competition or for self safety. If you need to reflect onconsideration on a way it too late. It is the idea of questioning without questioning.

Sparring

Ok we've had been given thru the first-rate and relaxed up and the approach part of the magnificence. The next a part of beauty typically is in which maximum human beings receives grew to turn out to be off of combined martial arts or grappling. It is the stay sparring portion of the elegance. This may be the maximum amusing trouble of sophistication for some or it can be the most dreaded portion. It is the challenge of the trainer to make it amusing for everybody. Remember you will have touch during this part of the beauty. You can sit down out some of the sparring, however you may ultimately have to take part. It is the teacher's system to make sure the partners are matched up lightly. It is likewise the technique of the instructor to keep the sparring at a a laugh pace. It is without a doubt easy for the sparring consultation to amplify to the volume of a combat. This is usually what turns off severa humans. No one ever wants to go to beauty and feature a few yahoo beat the crap out of you. You definitely need to depend upon the judgment of the teacher to make the beauty fun and secure.

You moreover have to be an first rate sparring accomplice. Sparring does now not ought to be a terrible problem. If you method sparring more like a recreation of tag than a sport of hit your associate with a brick, it's far going to be a good deal greater thrilling for each of you. Plus you may examine a lot extra from it. The days of guys bashing each others heads in are long beyond. Intelligent training need to be the order of the day. I moreover like situational sparring. This will come up with some appropriate abilities to each take gain of a scenario or educate you a manner to break out it.

There is a motion in Brazilian Jiu Jitsu that I truely be part of. It is the idea of Keep it Playful. There is a time at the same time as sparring and rolling turns into severe, but this is typically at the same time as there may be a combat coming up or a in form. Yes it is right enough to move a chunk more hard in elegance at instances, however it wants to be a mutual issue among each guys. Alright a few instructions will surrender with the sparring.

Cardio

Sparring is a awesome way to get into combating shape, but once in a while you need to add just a little greater cardio. So that is where I could throw approximately ten to fifteen minutes of cardio art work at the guys. It should commonly include 5 minute rounds with fantastic physical video games. It must include the whole lot from leap squats, to pushups, to perhaps even a few burpees. There are a few remarkable MMA sporting sports on YouTube. If you want to test out a few readymade workout routines, Bas Rutten and Georges St. Pierre have some notable exercising DVDs. I truely just like the Bas Rutten exercise absolutely as it comes with an audio CD. All you need to do is throw this in and it is going thru the exercise and also you don't want to watch a video show display. This quite plenty covers your everyday MMA or grappling elegance. Remember all teachers will educate a bit specific, however this could offer you with an idea on what to anticipate from a combined martial arts magnificence.

Etiquette

Having a critical set of policies for etiquette should be a given, however allow's in truth expect a few human beings had been raised by using wolves and don't have the essential not unusual experience to understand higher. This is not to offend everybody, however on occasion we genuinely want to be reminded of methods it need to be.

Chapter 10: Cleanliness

This want to be a smooth rule that each one people in this century should have mastered. But there are continuously exceptions to the rule of thumb of thumb. How typically have you ever been next to a person and that they fragrance like the incorrect surrender of 4 day vintage tuna sandwich? Ok permit's look at this to a martial arts magnificence, like blended martial arts or Brazilian jiu Jitsu. There is not something worse than being that man in magnificence. All you need to do is shower, and please placed on deodorant. It will make it an entire lot higher revel in for you and your accomplice. We used to have a man at the health club, wherein the alternative college students may additionally literally spray deodorant on the person as brief as his once more changed into became. Everyone modified into honestly too embarrassed to mention something to his face. This additionally goes for genuinely everyone who has a manual hard work challenge and is out within the warm temperature all day lengthy. Please bathe in advance than coming to splendor. Believe me anyone will appreciate the greater try.

Laundry

Let's stay at the hygiene and cleanliness kick. Please wash your clothes. Workout garments need to by no means be worn extra than as quickly as. When you get domestic after a difficult exercise consultation, take your sweaty clothes out of your tools bag. Next open your bag up so it is able to dry out. This will keep your device from starting to heady scent. One little trick I do as soon as I recognize I am going to be placing sweaty clothes in my fitness center bag is to take a small plastic bag to location them in. This maintains everything from soaking in all that sweat. You will recognize how horrible that is if you have ever left sweaty clothes in a fitness center bag for more than an afternoon or . It is in reality easy foul. You also can do this along side your jiu jitsu gi. Just placed it in the washing device and permit it soak. I usually don't dry my gi's. I normally hold them as plenty as dry.

Remember this is not pretty a extremely good deal the odor. If you do now not clean yourself and your clothes, it's far a breeding floor for all sorts of nasty germs. You can bypass around magnificence. These germs are one of the quickest strategies to close down a class. I've had multiple nasty bugs pass via my colleges and commands earlier than. We have had impetigo, ringworm, and the dreaded staph. One of the ideal strategies to save you the ones items is simple your self, your garments, and your tool.

I in my opinion hold a area of alcohol wipes in my gym bag. I wipe myself down right away after class. I always apprehend it may be as a minimum thirty mins to an hour earlier than I am able to take a tub after beauty. You also can use those alcohol wipes to wipe down all your device after class. Be advantageous to constantly wipe down boxing gloves, MMA gloves, shin guards, and head equipment. This will lessen down on germs. Just consider you bought the decision to the large show, and bam you could't fight or compete because of big nasty pores and pores and skin contamination. I can't provoke on you the want to lessen down on germ transmission, and who wants to roll with a person who smells and whose garments want to arise on their personal. Bottom line; wash your self and your device.

Foul Language

This have to moreover be a no-brainer. Try to hold foul language to a minimal. I understand it is easy to get round a set of guys and permit a few F bombs pass. Especially in the laid back environment of MMA or jiu Jitsu. Just consider someone's kids can also want to typically be there. In my colleges there were usually kids spherical. I may additionally not need a person's foul language round my youngsters so continuously maintain that during thoughts. Plus now not using foul language shows recognize in your teacher and in your faculty. Always count on that there are children at the mat and which have to take care of that. Remember you are notable heroes inside the ones children eyes. You are a position version to each toddler this is to be had in that faculty, whether or not or now not you're an instructor or a extremely-modern-day scholar. But if you anticipate it is OK to use foul language in front of toddler's perhaps you need to reevaluate a few things on your existence.

Never Call Out Your Instructor

One of the subjects I even have encountered in my years of teaching is there is constantly one man in each magnificence that wants to check the instructor. It is mostly a new guy. Someone who typically goes too tough whilst sparring and running on drills. It is in fact actually lousy form to call out the teacher. But I definitely have moreover found as an teacher you could't permit this arise. If you're the student you have to admire the teacher sufficient to no longer want to test your self in competition to him. In MMA and jiu Jitsu it's far not unusual for the teacher to spar and roll with university students. If I recognise I surely have the shape of fellows in elegance I will put on him completely out with drills and sparring, then offer him his hazard. Most instances simply the greater records from being the instructor is usually sufficient to make up the distinction, however once in a while it doesn't hurt to have a touch more side. In all the years I must normally tell while a student grow to be sorting out me. I actually have in no manner had a student without a doubt call me out, but I'm certain there are some accessible.

I may honestly have a take a seat down communicate with any scholar who did this. So the eliminate from this, is have a few apprehend in your instructor. Even in case you assume you may take him that is not the aspect. An teacher is there to train you, no longer to test your abilties as a fighter. This typically rings a bell in my memory of the vintage saying my dad used to mention. He knowledgeable me he taught me the whole thing I knew, however no longer the whole thing he knew.

Consistency

As an teacher one of the subjects I charge most in a student is how regular they came to elegance. This is so vital for optimum MMA or jiu Jitsu lessons. These training being greater non-traditional they typically in no way have the identical beauty attendance of the traditional martial arts schooling. So I commonly valued a pupil who need to show as tons as elegance regularly. This additionally includes showing up on time to elegance. I apprehend there are times even as you show up overdue to magnificence, however I absolutely have additionally visible university university students who is probably commonly past due to magnificence and pass over the incredible and comfortable-ups. If you will be past due extra than as soon as whether or not it is a way or university warfare with beauty times, please communicate with the teacher and let them recognize approximately it.

Another detail I usually appreciated from my college students is while they will call and allow me comprehend at the same time as they're no longer going to be in elegance. With the cutting-edge use of social media and smart phones, even a text or Facebook message can be high-quality. Just make certain your teacher in reality tests these things. Remember besides showing up on time, this moreover includes leaving early. This may be certainly as anxious on your trainer as showing up past due. I certainly have seen plenty of men who continually duck out early from magnificence so they don't ought to spar or do cardio art work. Get to elegance, get to elegance on time, stay for the entire elegance, if not talk together in conjunction with your instructor and permit them to recognize why. There is the vintage adage in the health company that as long as your buyers will pay it does not be counted in the event that they display up. Well as a martial arts instructor we need you to expose up as an entire lot as viable. We want to train you and it's miles a whole lot much less difficult to educate you in case you are there.

The Mat

In a blended martial arts or Brazilian jiu Jitsu splendor the mat is your private home. This is wherein you can spend most of you time at the same time as in splendor. The first factor you generally do earlier than stepping into the mat region is bow to the mat. This is a left over manner of lifestyles from the traditional martial arts, but it indicates appreciate to the college, the mat, and the instructor. The subsequent element to ensure you do is do not put on avenue footwear on any mat. Just maintain in mind that you going to be grappling and roll round on this mat. I can not stand to be rolling on a mat and revel in the grit of sand on the mat. I apprehend it's miles hard to keep a mat pristinely clean, however absolutely everyone has to do their factor. No footwear on the mat, is a terrific way to begin.

The subsequent goes again as a whole lot as the segment on cleanliness. You want to have, easy clothes, a easy gi, and a easy you. You have to recall that a hard and fast of sweaty humans rolling on a mat can be a amazing place to incubate all styles of germs. So be smooth. The mat is an important part of MMA or BJJ, appreciate it.

Cleaning the mat ground. Mats need to be swept regular and every so often in among commands. I experience that mats ought to be mopped every day. Then sometimes even between commands. I will give you an instance why. I changed into walking a MMA elegance at a nearby TKD college. My elegance became the very last commands of the day. So earlier than every beauty we had a ton of youngsters and adults taking walks anywhere inside the mats. Now this could be very regular for numerous faculties, but the TKD instructor was very lax on the opposite university university students wearing footwear at the mats and retaining it smooth. He have to mop the mats as fast as per week. So we began out out having a breakout of ringworm. We later determined out one of the youngsters inside the TKD splendor had some on his knee. The instructor did not save you him from schooling because of the truth they did no longer roll round on the mat and did not enjoy it become that crucial. We then began mopping the mats every day and being lots stricter on hygiene. As fast as this modified into installation location the prevalence of ringworm went down at once. Clean your mats every day. Clean the mats with Lysol or some component comparable. If your trainer does now not try this, ask if you could do it for him. I am positive he or she can also recognize the assist. It can be made actual easy with laptop virus sprayer complete of Lysol water and a reusable moist mop. Please do not use bleach. I definitely have visible it escape an entire beauty of children in pink pores and pores and skin burns. Sweat and dirt breed some quite funky stuff. Trust me.

Sparring

This is occasionally a very hard issue for a ultra-modern pupil. Keeping with the etiquette detail, sparring comes up lots. Some guys robotically comprehend a way to behave while sparring. Some men should be showed the proper way to spar. Then some guys have to have the proper manner beaten into their heads. It is continuously the technique of the instructor to set the right tone for any sparring session. Sparring is ready studying. Sparring isn't about beating the crap from your companions. I actually have seen such a lot of sparring instructions end up all out fights. It can get very ugly very speedy.

These are a few topics to hold in mind at the same time as sparring. First issue continually shake palms alongside facet your companion. Your companion could make this an excellent analyzing enjoy or a horrible one. The subsequent aspect is live with some thing drill your teacher has installation. If that may be a free sparring consultation use this time to prepare the whole thing you have been analyzing in elegance. If it is a limited consultation maintain on with the drills you are operating on. Nothing is greater stressful as a associate that if the person you're walking with will now not stay on challenge.

The next aspect to recollect is maintain the aggression levels down. This isn't always a combat. It is a sparring session. Yes sometimes sparring training get heated, but it isn't always a fight. Most times in case you preserve your aggression down, your companion can also moreover. This is usually better for learning. Once you want to guard yourself like you're in a combat, your mind shuts off the analyzing thing and switches to combat mode. If your accomplice is going manner too tough, actually ask him to take it easy. Most men after they recognize that they will be going to tough will go into reverse a hint. If they don't really inform him that may be a sparring consultation no longer a combat. Let them apprehend you are there to take a look at not fight. Even the most knock down drag out sparring consultation remains that, a sparring consultation. But then undergo in thoughts it's far a sparring consultation so you could probably take a punch or kick. You might also additionally get rolled and tapped out. This is a part of it. Even with managed sparring someone may also get harm. That is what makes sparring hard for some human beings.

I without a doubt have visible many guys simply not be capable of take a hard grappling consultation or a hard sparring consultation. I sincerely have additionally found that the excellent way to really get specific at a combat endeavor is through contact sparring. It doesn't want to be each day, however you do need to spar to appearance what method works, to get your range, and to get your timing. Sparring may be a fun factor, so simply consider to admire your accomplice and the elegance. Don't get too competitive and cope with each consultation as a way to examine some element. One of the exquisite methods to do that is what's referred to as in Brazilian Jiu Jitsu circles to go along with the flow roll. Flow rolling is an agreed upon sparring session wherein each men may have some offer and take. It is the agreed upon notion that you may now not strength out holds or be terrific competitive. This can be finished with upward push up furthermore. I revel in like this is one of the pleasant strategies to without a doubt get a hold close on timing and positioning. Most standup sparring isn't always completed like this. I actually have seen it to frequently decorate to an all out brawl. This is the time even as the teacher have to virtually paintings on education guys a manner to spar with out injuring their companions. It does no tremendous to knock out your sparring companion. Especially if one guys is in fact seeking to artwork on topics and the alternative is being an animal anywhere within the vicinity. I continuously try and improve pace, however not strength with the standup sparring. You should be capable of spar and by no means clearly experience the outcomes of the punches or kicks in some time. It is the drift rolling mentality transferred to the rise up. It is go with the flow sparring. I am no longer announcing don't contact every precise, however consider it greater like you are sparring together at the side of your youngster sister. You need the punches to be there but you don't need to take her head off. The men I see in jiu Jitsu beauty that generally have a wonderful draw near in this are the colored belts. But it virtually takes lots of the right education to get men to try this with their upward thrust up. So instructors stay on top of the sparring durations, cause them to gaining knowledge of sessions. Instruct them to spar with reading in mind. Teach them a way to research. Sparring is a pastime of tag. Not tag and overwhelm your cranium.

Chapter 11: Talking and Horseplay

Now don't get me incorrect I definitely have in no manner ran a completely strict beauty, but one component I do need from my college students is to pay hobby and no longer strive to speak over me on the same time as I am demonstrating or teaching some element in class. As a scholar this is your obligation to at least be quiet and respectful even as the instructor is speakme. Remember it's far adequate to speak in your companion whilst you walking on drills or techniques, however in case you are taking a ways from her or him studying you then are doing them a massive disservice. I in reality have visible guys, specially guys that have been in elegance for a while, do a drill a few instances then stop and talk for the rest of the time till it is time to the subsequent drill. This has commonly afflicted me. Please as a scholar art work on the drills in the allocated time you're there. It devices a totally lousy example to the contemporary guys in splendor to assume it's far adequate to forestall and socialize sooner or later of splendor. Like I said I am no longer great strict on my classes, however doing the art work ultimately of sophistication shows that a student wants to be there, and desires to studies.

The next is horseplay. I continuously idea of my coaching style mainly close to what I surely have visible from the Brazilian teachers. They are super laid again on the identical time as coaching instructions. The one issue I actually have located from schooling with Brazilian teachers is that you usually don't have severa talking or horseplay of their schooling. Horseplay in a MMA elegance or Jiu Jitsu beauty is always there, but please don't do it inside the direction of beauty. After elegance winds down is typically on the identical time as you spot the most horseplay, this is greater than Ok maximum of time. Remember those men are your fellow teammates and college college students don't permit it get out of hand and keep it splendid natured. Teasing is one thing bulling is a few other. Most people consider bulling as some element kids do. Bulling can seem to adults simply as easy as it can to youngsters. So an notable problem to do is usually just take a step lower back ask yourself if what you're doing will harm someone, physical and or emotionally. Keep each of these items in mind whilst you are in elegance or on the university. One of the high-quality sports activities is really maintain the horseplay all the way all the way down to a minimal. Think of class as even though it's miles a category you could have took in excessive university. You wouldn't snicker and shaggy canine tale while your math teacher turned into teaching. You trainer and companions will drastically appreciate it.

RESPECT

I can not stress this enough. Respect is one of the maximum primary human tenants. It is some element that is this kind of massive a part of the martial way. All martial arts whether or not or now not or not it's far a very conventional one, a bit a tremendous deal much less inflexible one like Brazilian Jiu Jitsu, or one like MMA, is constructed upon the idea of understand. It may be apprehend for your teacher. It can be recognize to your college. It can be recognize for your fellow classmates or recognize for yourself. Respect is a condition of honor. So to honor those assets you deliver recognize to them.

Following the primary etiquette steps above will let you honor them and by way of manner of the use of doing so indicates your apprehend for them. In my revel in, maximum all and sundry wants to be treated with admire. It is a very smooth hassle that may be so critical to 3 human beings. In my very very own career as a martial artist, I apprehend I grappled with the feeling of no longer being reputable as an instructor or as a competitor. I felt this specifically as soon as I changed into greater more youthful. It truly appears as I are getting older I don't enjoy the need to go looking that out as plenty as when I modified into extra younger. Respect is a palpable element. It can be felt nearly at once from a few people. Here is an clean manner to get understand from most human beings. Respect them. Talk to them as equals, shake their hand, examine their names, and be exceptional. It is an clean detail to do. Remember appreciate your instructor, your partners, your faculty, and most significantly your self. It will make your adventure inside the martial arts 1000 times more exceptional.

Fighter

A large a part of being a blended martial artist is being a fighter. Like I without a doubt have stated in advance it's miles tough to take MMA training and not be part of the fight element of combined martial arts. Whether you compete or not, being a blended martial artist is ready being a fighter. Just taking part in splendor makes you a fighter. I may not say that about the extra conventional martial arts like Tae Kwon Do or Karate. I accept as true with that doing those martial arts makes you a martial artist. It is a huge step from being a martial artist to being a fighter. Yes, on the same time as you educate in mixed martial arts you are a mixed martial artist, however you want to understand mixed martial arts are distilled conventional martial arts. The fat has been trimmed and all that is left is the sensible effective device. You don't have katas and or the opportunity nonessential subjects involved in the traditional martial arts.

Let me solution a few unique question earlier than it gets too a long way, most conventional martial arts had been at first supposed for stopping, consequently martial arts. Martial being of navy or warfare. A lot of them out of place their army factor and feature emerge as something else. The one problem that a few conventional martial arts do have that mixed martial arts are missing is the spiritual and philosophical elements. Now I am not speakme about religion. Religion and spirituality are absolutely various things. Being a fighter can suggest plenty of factors. We will just positioned it within the context of having the capability if one chooses so that you can get in a ring or a cage and fight. Remember there are masses more contexts to being a fighter, like shielding ones family and pals if want be. Being a fighter is a rustic of thoughts.

To be a fighter, a preference have to be made. The choice desires to be made if you are willing to threat your lifestyles to get proper into a cage or a ring. The choice desires to be made in case you are willing to offer your existence to defend your circle of relatives and friends. This sounds a touch over the pinnacle, but it's far one of the maximum sincere truths concerned in fight sports. You must be able to overcome this worry to be a fighter. Some men in no way even recognize that they bring about this fear. One of my preferred fighters, Enson Inoue, placed it splendid in an interview that you need to be willing to die each time you get within the cage. "Live as guy, Die as guy, grow to be a man", changed into the quote that caught with me. If you have got ever visible him fight, you'll see the resignation that he may not go away this cage. The legend goes that the Spartans had a pronouncing, "Come home collectively together with your guard or come domestic on it". This is how Inoue fought. I maintain a sure stage of admire for every fighter who enters a cage or a ring. It is something I can not provide an purpose of to a person who has not completed it. Competing in wrestling or grappling comes close to, but it lacks that element you feel competing in a MMA, boxing healthy, or kickboxing wholesome. Once one actually gets over the concern of stepping into the cage or ring you can definitely begin focusing on what it takes to be a MMA fighter. Once you have fought the whole lot else in life appears that masses easier. People don't appear the identical in some time. I grow to be in no way a huge man, but existence after the cage I am not often if ever intimidated thru some extraordinary person. You will see 100 strategies to interrupt someone down. Disputes at paintings or existence appear tame as quickly as you have got become a fighter.

We want to start out also pronouncing that it takes greater than a Tapout shirt and the balls to get inside the cage. I appreciate each person willing to get within the cage or the hoop, but it takes greater than that to be a actual fighter. It isn't always the fight that is the most hard a part of being a fighter, it's miles the education. I can't permit you to recognise how many of men I understand that say if they may fight and be competitive, but now not train they may fight each week. The education, the grind is in which a real fighter is born.

We will start first assuming you determined a train or a health club to begin your education. Remember it is able to be performed particular techniques, but if you need to win you find out a teach. As we stated in advance it does not must be a multimillion greenback facility. It simply has to give you the results you need. I even have constantly favored a small close knit institution. It appears to work better for me, being greater like a family. I definitely have worked out in larger gyms and it looks as if it changed into usually difficult to get the eye you want to grow as a fighter and get higher.

Ok you have got got the educate and you've the area to education consultation. The next issue you need to decide is how a good deal time you are inclined to place into turning into a fighter. If your purpose is to be a expert fighter, you may have to positioned the time in. Some country athletic commissions make fighters have a pleasant enormous kind of newbie fights earlier than they are in a position to show seasoned, and some don't. In Missouri you don't must have any wonderful amount of amateur fights. I do realize a few specialists which have lengthy past this course, but it has now not worked out properly for them. If you advise on being an beginner fighter and getting a few fights simply to see if you can do it, you will now not want close to the same amount of gym time as a seasoned fighter. I absolutely have coached dozens of fellows who handiest preferred to combat maybe one or fights. Just like within the movie Fightclub, you may never in reality realise your self till you have got been in a fight. These guys had a clear aim. They knew that had to mounted x quantity of labor to get in which they preferred to be.

The first at the list for each modified right into a health club and a train. I always advocate having a home base. I've visible guys wander from health club to health club in no manner in reality settling everywhere. This is extremely good to pick out up new competencies and spar with new people, but you need to a solid place in which you can not most effective have a look at, but refine your capabilities.

Next is identifying how tons time you may installed in your workout physical activities. I actually have coached some amazing varieties of men within the fitness center. I absolutely have had the exceptional proficient lazy man. This is the fellow who can get via on virtually his talent on my own. This guy works inside the fitness center, but first-class the bare minimal. The next is the splendid hard strolling man, who might not be first rate proficient, but works and does decorate. The final is the guy who works first rate tough and alternatives up the entirety like a sponge. This is the form of man if you advocated him doing leaping jacks could make him a higher jiu jitsu man; he may want to do them and start pulling off leaping jack passes. Then you have got were given the horrific soul who attempts the entirety to get higher, but simply doesn't seem to get it.

Ok allow's for a minute faux your college is open 7 days in step with week with lessons every hour. If you will be an newbie or a pro fighter you need to perform a little artwork at least six days in line with week. If you are starting out and want an clean schedule to comply with: a pair hours an afternoon for 3 days in keeping with week in elegance with a few type of aerobic or weight exercising on the times not in elegance. This is normally enough to get you in notable shape counting on how hard you are operating. A pinnacle robust hour exercise on the aerobic/weight days is generally actual sufficient. If you are a pro fighter you'll need to put in three-4 hours a day to get in all the belongings you desired. You need to work on grappling and putting approach. You will want grappling and standup sparring, and you'll furthermore need MMA sparring. I do accept as true with you best want one actual accurate sparring session in step with week lasting 1-2 hours.

Sparring needs to be tough, but now not with hard contact. Sparring stays a gaining knowledge of consultation, not a fight. This is a few factor all combatants need to analyze. It may be very smooth for a tough sparring session to turn right right into a fight. When this occurs nobody learns a few factor. This is one purpose you have to have a train. It is the coaches' machine to stop this from taking area.

Being a fighter is not easy whether or no longer it's far an novice or a pro fighter. It is a completely difficult, time consuming gadget. It is not an not possible technique. It takes a person who's committed. If you aren't willing to place in the time it's going to show on fight day. As a pro fighter that might be the distinction among paying the rent one month and no longer. There is so much art work that needs to be installation to be a a success fighter. Time in the health club is critical, however now not the best element that you need. The highbrow thing of being a fighter is as important or greater from time to time. If you aren't mentally in the fight it might be an extended night time for you on fight day.

Chapter 12: Mental Preparation

This has been the bane of many awesome gifted warring parties. I've visible guys that is probably international beaters fail to advantage their goals virtually at the reality that they will be no longer mentally prepared or mentally hard. Mental schooling isn't always a few component that you start at the same time as your combat camp begins. This is a manner of existence. Being a fighter isn't some component you turn on and turn off. If you try to technique your combat career this way, it's far going to be a sad one. Being a fighter is a lifestyle.

When I became no matter the reality that competing, the combat recreation occupied severa my time. I end up within the health club almost greater than I turned into at home. I furthermore worked a complete time task to guide my own family. When I may additionally want to come domestic I may want to spend hours on the laptop searching at fights, looking at technique films, or clearly studying video. It have become an obsession. Being a fighter is a attitude. It isn't approximately fancy techniques, it's far approximately building resilience. As they are saying it isn't about the punches you supply it's miles about how many you can take and hold transferring beforehand, to cite Rocky Balboa. This is what is called coronary coronary heart, however coronary heart is genuinely the mind-set to not forestall to hold transferring no matter what's thrown at you. This is the handiest underlying tendencies of the fighter mind-set. I've heard it in a million clichés, but most of them are accurate. The by no means say die attitude. Never surrender. As humans we've got an innate tendency while we are pushed we thrust back. We combat. Sometimes this is actually born in people and from time to time it may be cultivated in the fitness center. For some men it's far most effective a trade in self belief.

I've visible guys start off in the fitness center and take beating after beating. You might count on the ones guys don't have an oz.Of combat in them. But they preserve coming back. This is the primary sign of a fighter. It clearly sucks to return to the health club and feature your butt handed to you, even below the maximum managed occasions. I usually discovered that this could weed out maximum men. Being a fighter is difficult. It isn't best difficult bodily, however mentally. You without a doubt have to show off your ego, at the same time as you are becoming beat up on within the gymnasium. Here is a chance to appearance in case you are in an notable college. Does the man beating on you day in and day journey attempt that will help you get higher? If so, this is the manner you cultivate stopping spirit.

This will tell you if the guys in the health club are there for added than simply beating up on the amateur's. This is some thing I've constantly believed and tried to hold to my university college students. You can commonly beat up to your education partners, however if you don't forestall and make the effort to cause them to better, you could never get any better, due to the fact they may in no way get any better. The saying is going growing tides beautify all ships. This is why even inside the most hardcore MMA health club there needs to be a own family surroundings. If the men don't care about the opposite men in the gymnasium it isn't going to be a healthful region for growth as a fighter and as someone. This cultivation of fighting spirit helps you to construct and develop fighters and people. People with this preventing mind-set seem to do better in all aspects of their existence. I honestly agree with being a fighter has made my lifestyles higher.

As a fighter there are in fact things you need to mentally address. Between training and competition you cope with tension, exhaustion, home life, a assignment in case you are not competing entire time, and what I name health club lifestyles. Another aspect a few fighters need to address is EGO.

EGO

The ego of some opponents is so big you marvel how they're capable of healthful via any door. Ego is the inflated feeling of superiority to others. Some warring parties rely on this enjoy to mentally address the demanding conditions of preventing. I do apprehend it every so often requires a experience of invincibility to step within the cage. This can be a superb element, but also can be a opponents undoing. I definitely have labored with masses of guys who have been big fishes in their little ponds. Mainly because of the reality that that they had some success at one-of-a-kind sports activities sports or they had been the street preventing badass became wanna be fighter. I had a sign that hung over the door of my health club. Ego remains on the door or may be crushed out of you. I even have usually felt to grow to be a notable fighter or possibly a terrific fighter the ego preceding to beginning training had to be beaten, in order that they might be reborn and molded into their capability. It appears ego does no longer make a remarkable training companion

I really need to strain to more youthful up and coming combatants, lose the ego. It receives to your way. Confidence for your competencies is one problem. Over inflated chest thumping is a few element else. I without a doubt have seen hundreds men come in the health club thinking they're the baddest ape in the jungle. Most leave with their emotions harm and in no way come again, others comeback with handiest a touch plenty much less chest thumping each time. Like I said a sure amount of ego isn't always a awful difficulty, however I certainly have seen a loss destroy fighter's intellectual reputation and damage their fragile egos. Then ultimately harm their careers.

One of the first-rate matters for preserving men egos in take a look at is an exceedingly hard competitive crew. There isn't always anything like your training companions kicking the crap out of you on a each day basis. I even have felt this first hand and it's miles a humbling technique. Especially once I switched from entire time education expert to a recreational jiu jitsu participant. It is hard to preserve up with guys who teach two times an afternoon 5 to six days consistent with week. I now teach to 3 instances in keeping with week only as soon as an afternoon. So a piece butt kicking with certainly placed your ego in take a look at. But I revel in that may be a top notch trouble for a fighter. It will preserve you hungry to get better and to get in better shape. Being humble will make you a higher training companion, a better scholar, and in turn a higher fighter.

Anxiety

This may be a killer if not addressed properly. There is a difference between having real tension and having what's known as butterflies. Butterflies in advance than a competition are regular. It is not unusual to get a touch anxious and probable have some self doubt and horrible self talk. It comes again to our combating spirit; to compete you want to deal with this. Some men truly address this properly proper from the start.

There are a few matters that would honestly assist to cope with the tension of competing. The first component is experience. This inoculation to strain is one of the amazing tactics to get over some of the tension. Of course it comes another time to the antique seize 22 how do I get enjoy without having revel in. It is an smooth answer. You don't. So until you get enough experience you can ought to address the strain in remarkable techniques. One of the incredible strategies I even have determined to address tension spherical competing is to have a sturdy help device. This can be family resource or organization assist. If you have got had been given a terrific team they certainly are like a circle of relatives. Having unique human beings round you may virtually help take away the horrific self talk and doubt. This leads us to the following situation, family.

I actually have seen this difficulty, be the straw that breaks a fighter's lower lower back or the crutch that holds him up. When I began learning MMA and submission grappling, I grow to be very fortunate my first instruct became my dad. My dad have become an vintage school pro wrestler. He taught me approximately being a shooter. A shooter is a entice as trap can wrestling term for an completed submission grappler. I received't get into the data of capture wrestling, however it is a critically pleasing concern for any scholar of wrestling or submission wrestling. By having my dad as taken into consideration one in every of my first submission wrestling coaches, I have become a part of circle of relatives inside the health club and at home. This helped because of the fact I changed into capable of absolutely consider the understanding that he modified into passing alongside to me and I had his help. My dad has most effective ignored one in all my fights and has been to pretty much every healthy I surely have ever competed in. This kind of guide is so crucial.

As I had been given older I ultimately had been given married and had children of my very own. Having my dad in my corner modified into one hassle, however having your big others manual is a completely one-of-a-type animal. I actually have coached warring parties whose better halves and girlfriends did now not help their combat careers. It is form of no longer feasible for them to live advocated to educate and to combat. In the fourteen years I truely have coached fighters, I even have in no manner seen one guy be capable of stay with it with out the assist of their households. It is tough sometimes for wives and girlfriends to apprehend and to truly receive what it technique for a man to be a fighter, specially a entire time fighter. It takes sacrifice. It technique giving up pretty a few loose time that you may be spending with cherished ones. If you are not able to be an entire time fighter and want to art work a complete time technique it is even instances as tough. It in reality takes a certain shape of top notch super to be there and assist a fighter, in particular once they need to spend so much time a ways from own family. I had a string of girlfriends earlier than my wife that virtually did not recognize what it supposed, to be a fighter. To apprehend the determination it requires. I worked an 8-5 venture then is probably inside the gym till 9 nearly every night time. The girlfriends did no longer closing. My strength to be a blended martial artist outlasted them.

As I had been given older and my lady friend turned into my spouse, and our own family have been given huge, the stress of being a fighter took its toll. When you're single and don't simply have a circle of relatives to answer to and provide for, the fighter's life-style of regular education is not a actual trouble. You will generally have a massive different so that you may be part of it or now not. If you've got got one which makes you feel liable for spending time within the gym, it's miles actually a time to have a protracted speak about your desires or discover every other who will. This is the time whilst your enterprise in reality turns into your circle of relatives. If you've got were given a in reality pinnacle team you may emerge as spending a number of time with them. When you have got got were given crew buddies that actually care you may increase a exceptional strong bond. The real tough element is the problem retaining institution friends in a MMA setting. The training is tough and the hours are lengthy. This commonly keeps a quite constant turnover of guys at most MMA gyms.

Now permit's say you do have a partner and children. This is the time you'll should make some tough sacrifices near them. You will need to spend an entire lot of time some distance from them, except you're a complete time fighter. The problem is rarely any fighter may additionally need to make a dwelling as a entire time fighter in the beginning. A normal beginning fighter will make approximately $250 to expose for a combat and every other $250 to win a combat. So a possible $500 payday is probably hard to provide for a family. Trying to take even a combat a month is a completely hard and grueling way. The maximum I actually have ever visible become someone who had one five months in a row. His body was so beat up he took the following six months off absolutely to recover from the fights. So what I am announcing it's so tough to have a circle of relatives and fight complete time and paintings entire time. I would in no way say don't try it, however you need to keep your own family in balance.

If you begin with a loving supportive associate after which spend all of your time on the health club some distance from her she in all likelihood received't be supportive for that lengthy. If you do spend those extended hours far from own family you actually must make the time you do spend with them that rather more special. I appearance decrease decrease again on my time schooling and fighting and preference I must have realized the stress it places on relationships. I by no means had all people helping me with this stuff. This is one of the reasons I desired to put in penning this e-book changed into to help new men no longer make the equal errors that I did. I furthermore in no manner understood what I turned into missing in my child's lives. It is real easy to fall into the entice with a supportive accomplice, of questioning the entirety is probably proper sufficient and not putting in the try and make it top enough. I fell into this trap. I worked till 5 came domestic modified and may be out the door at 5:30 to be at my gym for the 6 o'clock class. I could then run instructions till 9pm. Clean and tidy up the health club and be home normally via way of nine:45. By this time my wife and son had been each in mattress. So in essence I observed them for 30 minutes a night time Monday thru Thursday. Then on the weekend I may usually run instructions on Saturday after which a few on Sunday. I modified into obsessed beyond belief.

I had a completely supportive partner so I in no manner felt like some thing have end up wrong. I modified into very incorrect. My partner stayed supportive, but it modified into hard on our relationship. It positioned stress have been there shouldn't have been strain. Plus I changed into lacking out on my son's life. My spouse spent almost 3 months inside the health facility in advance than the shipping of our son and I although spent most of my time at the gym chasing my dream. Chasing your dream can be very important, however don't allow the chase make you lose sight of what's simply vital. I allow her down no longer being there as a whole lot as I must had been. I experience the same manner about my son's first couple of years. I spent more time in the fitness center than with my son and my spouse.

This e-book isn't a dating guide, however take my advice, relationships take art work from both aspects. Mind the time you spend with your own family. I had a quite lousy damage prevent my MMA profession, so it gave me time with my family. It advanced the relationships with my partner and son. I have come to be capable of spend greater time with them. I will in no manner surrender being a fighter; I truly have a take a look at the manner I do topics lots in each different way. I now have a health club at my house wherein I do masses of my art work. My son is normally right there with me. For a 3 12 months vintage he desires to be in our fitness center an awful lot. I love having him in there with me. We name it the dog house. It is simplest a piece 20'x 20' constructing with mats and bags. I am not fighting, however I still teach regular or most days. Having this at home shall we me do the dull stuff like heavy bag paintings or lifting weights and I am only 50' from the house. I despite the fact that teach in BJJ, but that college is without a doubt 30 miles from my residence so I don't spend all my time there. I educate more than one days every week so I'm now not away too much. There are a pair of factors I could recommend about own family and preventing.

First discover a proper supportive huge other, due to the fact you'll ought to be some distance from your own family. Sit down and communicate about your desires together in conjunction with your circle of relatives. Plan a time desk. Communication is so crucial. Take this from a man who is incredible lousy with this simple skills. You need to with the aid of using the use of now be attending a college and have the colleges time desk. Next plan out it sluggish together collectively together with your own family.

Then get as masses device as you can for your own home. That manner you may do a whole lot of your primary conditioning type stuff for your very personal at your home. I recognize it's miles extremely good to visit elegance and do conditioning, however a number of the time you spend on the fitness center is probably spent at domestic. Especially when you have children, they'll imitate the property you do as a determine. Every time I'm within the ground doing pushups or sit down down-ups, my youngest son is right subsequent to me doing them proper along. That is a exquisite motivator. Do you need your children to look you finish and surrender?

www.ingramcontent.com/pod-product-compliance
Lightning Source LLC
Chambersburg PA
CBHW071444080526
44587CB00014B/1984